DNA AND RNA: PROPERTIES AND MODIFICATIONS, FUNCTIONS AND INTERACTIONS, RECOMBINATION AND APPLICATIONS

PROLINE

BIOSYNTHESIS, REGULATION AND HEALTH BENEFITS

DNA and RNA: Properties and Modifications, Functions and Interactions, Recombination and Applications

Additional books in this series can be found on Nova's website
under the Series tab.

Additional e-books in this series can be found on Nova's website
under the e-book tab.

Cell Biology Research Progress

Additional books in this series can be found on Nova's website
under the Series tab.

Additional e-books in this series can be found on Nova's website
under the e-book tab.

DNA AND RNA: PROPERTIES AND MODIFICATIONS, FUNCTIONS AND INTERACTIONS, RECOMBINATION AND APPLICATIONS

PROLINE

BIOSYNTHESIS, REGULATION AND HEALTH BENEFITS

BOUZID NEDJIMI
EDITOR

New York

For permission to use material from this book please contact us:
Telephone 631-231-7269; Fax 631-231-8175
Web Site: http://www.novapublishers.com

NOTICE TO THE READER

Additional color graphics may be available in the e-book version of this book.

Library of Congress Cataloging-in-Publication Data

ISBN: 978-1-62257-739-2

Library of Congress Control Number: 2012944807

Published by Nova Science Publishers, Inc. † New York

Contents

Preface

Proline might be the most studied amino acid in nature. Many authors have reviewed its many functions in cell homeostasis. Not only it is essential in primary metabolism, but it is also involved in cell defense response to a variety of stresses. This book presents topical research data in the study of proline functions, including role of proline in plant subject to salinity, proline cycle and its role in secondary metabolite accumulation, role of proline in catalyzing the asymmetric reaction, studies of polyproline peptides, structural characteristics and transition mechanisms of proline-rich peptides, functions of proline in behavior of neonatal chicks and tumor suppressor activities of proline oxidase.

Chapter I – Salinity affects many aspects of plant metabolism and the accumulation of various organic solutes that contribute to turgor maintenance. Among them, the accumulation of low molecular weight solutes, compatible osmolytes, such as proline are thought to function as osmoprotectants. Proline is a major organic osmolyte that accumulates in a variety of plant species in response to salinity stress. This amino acid has positive effects on osmotic adjustment, enzyme and membrane integrity in plants grown under stress conditions. In many, plant species exogenous applications of this amino acid can lead to significant increases in growth and final crop yield under salinity stress. This review focuses on proline production and accumulation in plants subject to salt stress, and successful applications of this compound for improving plant stress tolerance.

Chapter II – Proline is an amino acid that has been widely studied because of its multiple functions in plant cells. Accumulation of proline in response to different kinds of stress, such as drought, high salinity, UV irradiation and exposure to heavy metals is well documented. This amino acid has been described as exhibiting several functions in plant defense response, such as acting as a compatible osmolyte, having antioxidant properties and contributing to cell recovery after stress, among others. Besides its central role in defense response, the influence of proline in secondary metabolite accumulation has been a subject of research. Shetty and co-workers have proposed that the proline cycle could be coupled to the pentose phosphate pathway (PPP), an important metabolic route that generates erithrose-4-phosphate. The latter compound is the precursor of the shikimate pathway, whose end-product (chorismate) becomes the branch point between primary and secondary metabolism and can lead to the synthesis of important secondary metabolites. In the model proposed by Shetty, proline synthesis from glutamate generates two molecules of $NADP^+$, which act as cofactors of the first two enzymes in the PPP. Stimulating the proline cycle of biosynthesis and degradation could induce the PPP and generate an excess of erythrose-4-phosphate, thereby, driving the carbon flux towards the shikimate pathway. In our work, the authors intend to review the effect of stimulating proline cycle on the accumulation of secondary metabolites, by the addition of proline analogs or precursors. Regarding this subject, the authors are going to discuss our findings related to anthraquinone production in *Rubia tinctorum* cell suspension cultures. Beside this, the authors will analyze the role of proline cycle in the defense response, focusing on its antioxidant activity and the effect on the final accumulation of secondary metabolites.

Chapter III – A few new prolinethioamide compounds, designed and prepared from readily available natural amino acid L-proline and L-valine, have been found to be active catalysts for the direct aldol reaction of various aldehydes with acetone, cyclohexanone or cyclopentanone at 0°C or rt. Using only 2 mol% or 0.2 mol% loading of organocatalysts 1 or 2, the reaction could give high enantioselectivity with up to 96% enantiomeric excess for the reaction of 2-nitrobenzaldehyde with acetone or higher than 99% ee for the reaction of 3-nitrobenzaldehyde with acetone in aqueous media, respectively. Moreover, using the simple dipeptide derivative 3, the authors unexpectedly found the different regioselectivity product, 1,2-diol and 1,4-diol, could be achieved with high yields and high enantioselectivities in the reaction of hydroxyl acetone and aromatic aldehydes promoted by the different additives at room temperature. Summarily, these structurally simple catalysts have been proven to be highly efficient prolinethioamide derivatives in asymmetric aldol reaction. In addition, the authors also explored a few known organocatalysts derived from L-proline application for some organic reaction. For example, the L-proline 4 has been found that it can catalyze well the ring-opening of epoxide with allylmetal reagent. And the catalyst 5 could promote the asymmetric allylation of aldehyde. The N-oxide compound 6 could effectively catalyze the ring-opening of epoxide and halide atom donor. The organophophine compound 7 is a highly efficient catalyst in the asymmetric Michael reaction of chalcone and cyclohexanone in our work. Our further work would mainly focus on the design and synthesis of polymer-supported L-proline or L-proline derivatives with tunable morphology. And the relationship between the structure and catalytic activity of these catalysts would also be investigated.

Chapter IV – Polyproline-II (PPII) helix is a very common regular pattern in proteins. It is observed in many protein structures, and is considered to be an important transient structure in Intrinsically Disordered Proteins. This structure is also part of the recognition element for the SH3 domains, which are an essential element for signal transmission into the cell. While numerous studies and models have been made on this structure, a detailed understanding of the PPII helices behavior is still lacking. The aim of this chapter is to explore this structure by different biophysical approaches, in order to improve the PPII model available. A series of polyproline peptides of varying lengths from 3 to 20 were studied by NMR. Hydrodynamics parameters such as diffusion coefficients were measured. These values were interpreted in terms of the fractal dimension, an hydrodynamic value evaluating the interaction between a molecule and the solvent. This analysis confirms that the PPII helix is indeed an extended and rigid structure. However, it was shown that a minimum of 6 sequential prolines are needed and that shorter proline stretches do not display a full PPII pattern. Moreover, diffusion coefficient measures were compared to calculations obtained by several diffusion models. It appears that most of these models, developed for the general case, are not well adapted to PPII helices and are not always able to provide results close to the experimental values. Some trends appear from this comparison nonetheless, and it is found that molecular models seem better suited to describe PPII helices than continuous models. Finally, the authors generated several thousands of PPII helix conformers by varying the dihedral angles around the canonical values, as well as generating a given amount of cis prolines. This ensemble of conformers was then used as a pattern to evaluate the effect of cis-proline on the measure. All these results help creating a complete overview of PPII helices but also stress that biophysical methods would certainly be one of the best ways of studying this kind of biological patterns.

Chapter V – In this chapter, the authors are interested in relatively small proline-rich peptides that in spite of their apparent simplicity have generated considerable controversy in the literature. First, the authors explore issues related to the conformational space of pure polyproline (PP) peptides. PP peptides are generally associated with two well-characterized helical structures: (a) a left-handed polyproline helix (PPII), with all peptide bonds in the transisomer conformation; and (b) a more compact right-handed polyproline helix (PPI), with all the peptide bonds in the cis-isomer conformation. Because of their relatively rigid structure, PPII peptides have been used as a "molecular ruler" in structural biology, especially for the validation of spectroscopic rulers in F¨oster resonance energy transfer. However, recent experimental and theoretical studies have called this traditional picture of polyproline peptides as a "rigid rod" into question, since PP peptides in aqueous solution display static structural heterogeneity with subpopulations of different end-to-end distances that do not interconvert on the time scales of nano- to milliseconds. Second, the authors investigate the properties of guest amino acids in host proline peptides. Experimentally, there has been considerable emphasis on deriving an "intrinsic PPII propensity" scale for amino acids in a proline-rich host-guest environment, in order to understand the role of PPII conformations in denatured proteins. In particular, Circular Dichroism (CD) experiments attribute a high PPII propensity to several amino acids, a claim that has been disputed by theoretical work. In order to probe these issues, the authors have used classical molecular dynamics (MD) simulations, with state-of-the-art force fields and novel sampling methodology to study the free energy landscapes, conformational characteristics and equilibrium populations of pure PP peptides of various lengths in different environments and of proline-based oligopeptides with single and multiple guest amino acids. Our results point to the presence of many free energy minima associated with stable or metastable PP structures, which are characterized in terms of the cis/trans pattern of the prolyl bonds. The authors have also characterized several mechanisms for the interconversion between PPI and PPII structures. For the host-guest systems, the authors find no evidence for an intrinsic PPII propensity in any of the guest amino acids other than proline. Instead, the PPII content as derived from experiments may be explained in terms of: (i) a local correlation between the dihedral angles of the guest amino acid and the proline residue immediately preceding it; and (ii) a non-local correlation between the cis/trans states of the peptide bonds. In terms of the latter, the authors find that the presence of a guest (other than proline, tyrosine or tryptophan) increases the trans content of most of the prolyl bonds, which results in an effective increase of the peptide PPII content.

Chapter VI – Proline is formally an imino acid, but is usually called an amino acid. It is not an essential amino acid, since proline is biosynthetically derived from the amino acid L-glutamate. Food intake was mildly stimulated by low levels of intracerebroventricular (i.c.v.) injection of L-proline, but was suppressed by high levels in chicks. L-Proline was decreased in the telencephalon and diencephalon under several different stressors including restraint with isolation-induced and fasting stress. Central L-proline induced sedative and hypnotic effects in a dose-dependent manner, suggesting that L-proline may have an important role in attenuating the stress response in the central nervous system of chicks. The central effects of L-proline, D-proline and *trans*-4-hydroxy-L-proline were investigated by using the acute stressful model with neonatal chicks. Sedative and hypnotic effects were induced by all compounds, while plasma corticosterone release under isolation stress was only attenuated by L-proline. To clarify the mechanism by which L-proline and D-proline induce sedative and hypnotic effects, the contribution of the strychnine-sensitive glycine receptor (glycine receptor) and *N*-methyl-D-aspartate glutamate receptor (NMDA receptor) were further investigated. The glycine receptor antagonist strychnine was co-injected i.c.v. with L-proline or D-proline. The suppression of isolation-induced stress behavior by D-proline was attenuated by strychnine. However, the suppression of stress behavior by L-proline was not attenuated. The NMDA receptor antagonist (+)-MK-801 was co-injected i.c.v. with L-proline. The suppression of stress behavior by L-proline was attenuated by (+)-MK-801. These results indicate that L-proline and D-proline differentially induce sedative and hypnotic effects through NMDA and glycine receptors, respectively. Using microdialysis, the effect of L-proline on monoamine release in the medio-rostral neostriatum /hyperstriatum ventrale (MNH) of freely moving and restricted chicks was investigated. A 30 min handling stress resulted in significant increases of extracellular homovallinic acids (HVA), a dopamine metabolite, and 5-hydroxyindoleacetic acid (5-HIAA), a serotonin metabolite, in the MNH. L-Proline, perfused through a microdialysis probe in the MNH during the stressed condition, significantly attenuated the average dialysate concentration of HVA produced by handling-stress. Handling-stress resulted in a significant increase in 5-HIAA levels in the control group, which were attenuated by profusion with L-proline. These results show that perfusion of L-proline decreased the release of dopamine and serotonin in the MNH caused by handling-stress.

Chapter VII – Proline oxidase (POX) is a p53-regulated redox gene that mediates tumor suppression by inducing cell cycle arrest and proline-dependent apoptosis. A degenerate p53 consensus binding site in the POX promoter allows the gene to respond to p53. POX functions as a mitochondrial tumor suppressor by inducing intrinsic and extrinsic apoptosis, mediating a G2 cell cycle arrest, and reducing hypoxia-inducible factor (HIF) signaling. Consistent with its role as a tumor suppressor, POX expression levels are frequently much lower in renal, colorectal, pancreatic, liver, and stomach tumor tissues than in their normal tissue counterparts. The loss of POX is not due to genetic or epigenetic mechanisms but instead occurs through upregulation of the mir-23b microRNA, which suppresses translation of POX mRNA by binding to its 3' untranslated region. P53-induced POX generates reactive oxygen species (ROS) through oxidation of proline. Pyrroline-5-carboxylate, the product of proline oxidation, is recycled back to proline with redox transfers or converted to glutamate and a-ketoglutarate; the latter enhances the prolyl hydroxylation of HIF and its proteasomal degradation. POX mediates the activation of the NFAT transcription factor by p53 through activation of the calcium/calmodulin-dependent phosphatase, calcineurin. POX-induced ROS mobilizes calcium from intracellular stores to activate calcineurin, which then activates the NFAT transcription factor to modulate gene expression and apoptosis. The initiation of calcineurin-regulated transcription factor pathways may affect gene expression events important in not only apoptosis but other p53-regulated physiological processes. POX also mediates p53-independent signaling pathways. Peroxisome proliferator-activated receptor ligands mediate apoptosis in human lung cancers by inducing POX. Upregulation of POX expression dramatically decreases phosphorylation of MEK and ERK, which is partially reversed by expression of manganese superoxide dismutase. Overexpression of a constitutively active form of MEK suppressed POX-induced apoptosis, suggesting the involvement of MEK/ERK signaling and further confirming the role of ROS/superoxides in POX-induced apoptosis. Etoposide, a conventional anticancer drug, upregulates p53, POX, NFAT, and ROS, and induces apoptosis, in responsive tumor cells. The involvement of POX in both p53-dependent and -independent tumor suppressor pathways makes it an attractive strategic target for cancer therapy in a variety of human cancers.

In: Proline
Editor: Bouzid Nedjimi

ISBN: 978-1-62257-739-2

Chapter I

Involvement of Proline in Plant Response to Salt Stress

Nedjimi Bouzid [*]

Laboratoire d'Exploration et Valorisation des Ecosystèmes Steppiques, Université de Djelfa, Faculté des Sciences de la Nature et de la Vie, Djelfa, Algérie

Abstract

Salinity affects many aspects of plant metabolism and the accumulation of various organic solutes that contribute to turgor maintenance. Among them, the accumulation of low molecular weight solutes, compatible osmolytes, such as proline are thought to function as osmoprotectants. Proline is a major organic osmolyte that accumulates in a variety of plant species in response to salinity stress. This amino acid has positive effects on osmotic adjustment, enzyme and membrane integrity in plants grown under stress conditions. In many, plant species exogenous applications of this amino acid can lead to significant increases in growth and final crop yield under salinity stress. This review focuses on proline production and accumulation in plants subject to salt stress, and successful applications of this compound for improving plant stress tolerance.

---

[*] Dr. Nedjimi Bouzid. Université de Djelfa, Faculté des Sciences de la Nature et de la Vie, Cité Aîn Chih, BP 3117 Djelfa 17000, Algérie. Tel.: + 213 662 128 131. Fax: + 213 27 900 201. E-mail address: bnedjimi@yahoo.fr

Keywords: Amino acid, Osmolyte, Proline, Salt stress, Osmotic adjustment

Abbreviations

P5CS: Pyrroline-5-carboxylate synthetase; P5CR: Pyrroline-5-carboxylate reductase.

1. Introduction

Among the environmental stresses, salt stress is one of the most adverse factors of plant growth and productivity (Nedjimi, 2011b). Plants are subjected to several environmental stresses that adversely affect growth, metabolism, and yield. Salinity, drought, extreme temperatures, heavy metals and radiation are the important stress factors limiting the productivity of crops (Reddy et al., 2004).

Salt stress tolerance is seen in almost all plant species but its extent varies from species to species. Although the general effects of salinity on plant growth are fairly well known, the primary effects of salt stress at the biochemical and the molecular levels are not well understood (Lutts et al., 1999; Ashraf and Foolad, 2007).

Despite the presence of a strong correlation between stress tolerance and accumulation of proline in higher plants, in other plants subject to salinity, accumulation of proline was deemed to be a symptom of salt injury rather than an indication of salt tolerance (Ashraf and Foolad, 2007). Lutts et al. (1999) found that proline did not take part in osmotic adjustment in salt stressed rice and its accumulation seemed to be a symptom of injury rather an indicator of salt tolerance.

In order to improve the agricultural productivity within the limited land resources, it is imperative to ensure higher crop yields against salt stress. Understanding plant responses to salinity is of great importance and also a fundamental part for making the crops salinity tolerant. In this article, we provide an overview of the current understanding of proline production and metabolism under salt stress. In addition, we will describe the applications of these compounds to improve plant stress.

Many plants cope with osmotic stress by synthesizing and accumulating some compatible solutes, which are termed as osmoprotectants or osmolytes. These compounds are small, electrically neutral molecules, which are non-toxic even at molar concentrations (Ashraf and Foolad, 2007). During osmotic stress, plant cells accumulate solutes to prevent water loss and to reestablish cell turgor. The solutes that accumulate during the osmotic adjustment include ions such as K^+, Na^+, and Cl^- or organic solutes that include nitrogen-containing compounds, such as proline and other amino acids, polyamines and quaternary ammonium compounds like glycine betaine (Ashraf and Harris, 2004). The organic solutes are compatible with cellular processes and accumulate to high levels in the cytosol with increasing salinity.

Production of osmolytes is a general way to stabilize membranes and maintain protein conformation at low leaf water potentials. The synthesis and accumulation of osmolytes varies among plant species as well as among different cultivars of the same species. Osmolytes play a major role in osmotic adjustment and also protect the cells by scavenging ROS (Chris et al., 2006).

Proline is also known to be involved in reducing the photodamage in the thylakoid membranes by scavenging and/or reducing the production of superoxide radicals (O_2^-). Proline accumulation in plants is caused, not only by the activation of proline biosynthesis, but also by the inactivation of proline degradation, thereby resulting in a decrease in the level of accumulated proline in rehydrated plants. Proline degradation to glutamic acid via pyrroline-5-carboxylate in higher plants is catalyzed by proline dehydrogenase and pyrroline-5-carboxylate dehydrogenase in mitochondria (Reddy et al., 2004).

In the presence of low water potentials, the accumulation of compatible osmolytes, involved in osmoregulation allows additional water to be taken up from the environment, thus buffering the immediate effect of water shortage within the plant. Therefore, the high level of proline enabled the plant to maintain low water potentials. Besides this, proline also serves as a sink for energy to regulate redox potentials, as a hydroxyl radical scavenger and acts as a storage compound and nitrogen source for rapid growth after stress (Simiroff and Cumbes, 1989). It has been reported that proline alleviates NaCl stress induced enhancement in oxygenase and carboxylase activities of Rubisco (Sivakumar et al., 2000).

Proline accumulation is one of the adaptations of plants to salinity and water deficit (Nedjimi et al., 2006; Misra and Gupta, 2005) (Figure 1). It has also been widely advocated that proline accumulation uses as parameter of selection for salt stress tolerance (Levignron et al., 1998). However, some authors consider enhanced proline level merely a stress effect, rather than a cause of stress to tolerance. Recently, it has been reported that proline accumulation appears to be a reaction of salt stress damage and not a plant response associated with salt tolerance (Lutts et al., 1999).

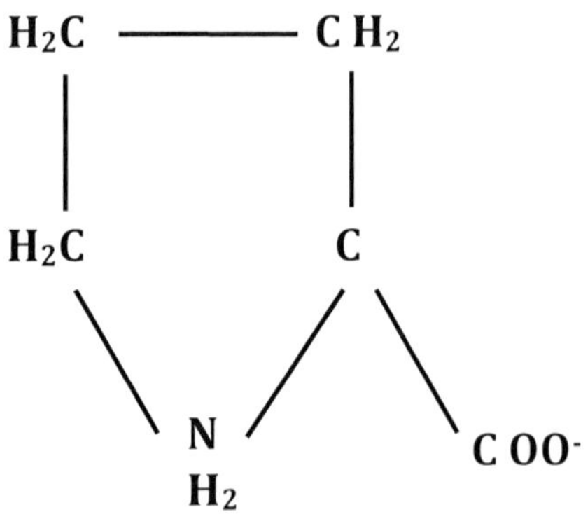

Figure 1. L-Proline.

2. Proline Production and Accumulation in Salt Stressed Plants

In response to salinity stress in plants, proline accumulation normally occurs in the cytosol where it contributes substantially to the cytoplasmic osmotic adjustment (Nedjimi, 2011c).

The accumulation of proline under stress protects the cell by balancing the osmotic pressure of cytosol with that of vacuole and external environment (Gadallah, 1999). In addition to their role as cytosolic osmotytica, this solute may interact with cellular macromolecules such as enzymes and stabilize the structure and function of such macromolecules (Misra and Gupta, 2005). Proline accumulation may contribute to osmotic adjustment at the cellular level. Many investigators have were demonstrated the osmoprotective role of proline at the whole plant level and in cell cultures (Nedjimi and Daoud, 2006; Nedjimi, 2011b). At genetic level, it has been demonstrated that proline accumulation under salt stress by bacterial gene, engineered into plant and resulting in proline over production can also increase ability to tolerate salinity. The accumulation of proline oxidation or decreased incorporation of proline into protein due to impaired protein synthesis and reduced growth. The increased or decreased regulation of enzymes of proline metabolism in response to stress has ben demonstrated in many varieties of crop species (Misra and Gupta, 2005). In plants, the precursor for proline biosynthesis is glutamic acid. Two enzymes, pyrroline-5-carboxylate synthetase (P5CS) and pyrroline-5-carboxylate reductase (P5CR), play major roles in proline biosynthetic pathway (Delauney and Verma,

1993) (Figure 2). The increase in proline content under salt stress may be correlated with the increased synthesis of P-5-C reductase and glutamyl kinase activity and low activity of the degrading enzyme, proline oxidase. Proline accumulation under salt stress can be explained by the higher inhibitory rate of proline oxidase. P5CR, a key enzyme catalyzes the reaction from glutamate to proline. P5CR activity has been shown to increase under salt stress (Ashraf, 1994). Proline accumulation is increased in presence of salinity may, therefore, be due to increased production of P5C, which is then converted to proline by normal or enhanced level of P5CR activity (Misra and Gupta, 2005).

Proline is known to occur widely in higher plants and normally accumulates in large quantities in response to salt stresses (Nedjimi et al., 2006; Nedjimi and Daoud, 2006). In addition to its role as an osmolyte for osmotic adjustment, proline contributes to stabilizing sub-cellular structures (e.g. membranes and proteins), scavenging free radicals, and buffering cellular redox potential under stress conditions. It may also function as a protein compatible hydrotrope (Ashraf and Foolad, 2007; Mansour, 1998), alleviating cytoplasmic acidosis, and maintaining appropriate $NADP^+$/NADPH ratios compatible with metabolism (Hare et al., 1999). Furthermore, proline is known to induce expression of salt stress responsive genes, which possess proline responsive elements in their promoters (Ashraf and Foolad, 2007).

Table 1. Summary of the effects of salt stress on proline acumulation on different plant species

Plant Species	Family	Reference
Atriplex halimus	Chenopodeaceae	Nedjimi et al. (2006)
Phaseolus vulgaris	Fabaceae	Jiménez-Bremont et al. (2006)
Haloxylon persicum	Chenopodeaceae	Song et al. (2006)
Hordeum vulgare	Poaceae	Ueda et al. (2007)
Juncus kraussii	Juncaceae	Naidoo and Kift (2006)
Allium cepa	Amaryllidaceae	Mansour (1998)
Oryza sativa	Poaceae	Hien et al. (2003)
Plantago crassifolia	Plantaginaceae	Vicente et al. (2004)
Kochia prostrata	Chenopodeaceae	Karimi et al. (2005)
Salsola dendroides	Chenopodeaceae	Heidari-Sharifabad and Mirzaie-Nodoushan (2006)
Sorghum bicolor	Poaceae	Lacerda et al. (2005)
Salvadora persica	Salvadoraceae	Maggio et al. (2000)
Setaria italica	Poaceae	Veeranagamallaiah et al. (2007)
Triticum aestivum	Poaceae	Wang et al. (2007)
Lycopersicon esculentum	Solanaceae	Claussen (2005)

Accumulation of proline under salt stress in many plant species has been correlated with stress tolerance, and its concentration has been shown to be generally higher in stress-tolerant than in stress-sensitive plants (Table 1.)

Besides positive effects of proline on improving plant salt tolerance at the organismal level, considerable improvement in salt tolerance has also been observed at the cellular level (Ashraf and Foolad, 2007).

3. Exogenous Application of Proline to Salt Stressed Plants

Exogenous application of proline caused osmoprotection and enhanced growth in many plant species growing under saline conditions (Kaya et al., 2007). In bean, exogenous application of proline counteracted the adverse effects of salinity seedling growth (Demir and Kocaçalişkan, 2002). In melon culture under saline conditions, exogenous application of proline resulted in a decrease in Na^+ accumulations and an increase in growth, K^+ and N (Kaya et al., 2007). Exogenous supply of proline to stressed plants of *Vicia faba* increased their growth (Gadallah, 1999). Also exogenous application of proline increased activities of superoxide dismutase and peroxidase, which normally contribute to increased salt tolerance in plants subject to salinity (Ashraf and Foolad, 2007).

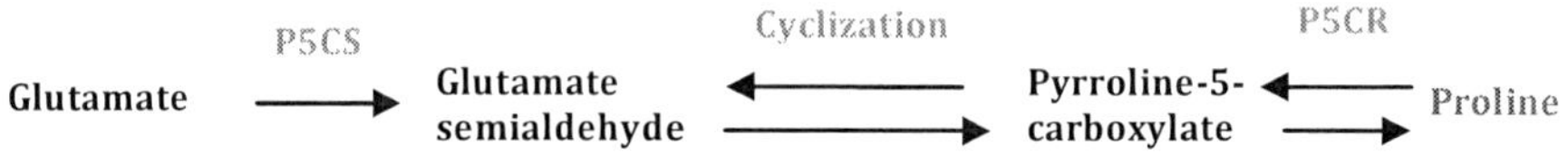

Figure 2. Biosynthetic pathway of proline in higher plants (Ashraf and Foolad, 2007).

Conclusion

Proline, which occurs widely in higher plants, accumulates in larger amounts than other amino acids in salt stressed plants. This compound is thought to play adaptive roles in mediating osmotic adjustment and protecting cellular structures in stressed plants. Exogenous application of proline to stressed plants was applied to increase the concentrations of this compound in plants grown under stress conditions to increase their stress tolerance.

Acknowledgments

Algerian Ministry of Higher Education and Scientific Research is gratefully acknowledged (Project no. F–02820100012).

References

Ashraf M., (1994) Breeding for salinity tolerance in plants, *Crit. Rev. Plant Sci.* 13: 17–42.

Ashraf M., Harris P.J.C. (2004) Potential biochemical indicators of salinity tolerance in plants. *Plant Sci.* 166: 3–16.

Ashraf, M., Foolad M.R. (2007) Roles of glycine betaine and proline in improving plant abiotic stress resistance. *Environ. Exp. Bot.* 59:206–216.

Chris A., Zeeshan M., Abraham G., Prasad S.M. (2006) Proline accumulation in *Cylindrospermum sp*. Environ. Exp. Bot. 57:154-159.

Claussen W. (2005) Proline as a measure of stress in tomato plants. *Plant Sci.* 168: 241-248.

Delauney, A.J., Verma, D.P.S., (1993) Proline biosynthesis and osmoregulation in plants. *Plant J.* 4: 215–223.

Demir Y., Kocaçalişkan I. (2002) Effect of NaCl and proline on bean seedlings cultured in vitro. *Biol. Plant.* 45:597– 599.

Gadallah M.A.A. (1999) Effect of proline and glycinebetaine on *Vicia faba* responses to salt stress. *Biol. Plant.* 42: 247–249.

Hare, P.D., Cress,W.A., van Staden, J., 1999. Proline synthesis and degradation: a model for elucidating stress-related signal transduction. *J. Exp. Bot.* 50 : 413–434.

Heidari-Sharifabad H., Mirzaie-Nodoushan H. (2006) Salinity-induced growth and some metabolic changes in three *Salsola* species. *J. Arid Environ.* 67:715–720.

Hien D.T., Jacobs M., Angenon G., Hermans C., Thu T.T., Son L.V., Roosens N.H. (2003) Proline accumulation and Δ^1-pyrroline-5-carboxylate synthetase gene properties in three rice cultivars differing in salinity and drought tolerance. *Plant Sci.* 165: 1059-1068.

Jiménez-Bremont J.F., Becerra-Flora A., Hernández-Lucero E., Rodríguez-Kessler M., Acosta-Gallegos J.A, Ramírez-Pimentel J.G. (2006) Proline accumulation in two bean cultivars under salt stress and the effect of polyamines and ornithine. *Biol. Plant.* 50 (4): 763-766.

Karimi G., Ghorbanli M., Heidari H., Khavari Nejad R.A., Assareh M.H. (2005) The effects of NaCl on growth, water relations, osmolytes and ion content in *Kochia prostrata*. *Biol. Plant.* 49(2): 301–304.

Kaya C., Tuna A.L., Ashraf M., Altunlu H. (2007) Improved salt tolerance of melon (*Cucumis melo* L.) by the addition of proline and potassium nitrate. *Environ. Exp. Bot.* 60: 397-403.

Lacerda C.F., Cambraia J., Oliva M.A., Ruiz H.A. (2005) Changes in growth and in solute concentrations in *Sorghum* leaves and roots during salt stress recovery. *Environ. Exp. Bot.* 54: 69–76.

Levigneron A., Lopez F., Vansyuyt G., Berthomieu P., Fourcroy P., Casse-delbart f. (1995) Les plantes faces au stress salin. *Cahiers Agri.* 4: 263–273.

Lutts, S., Majerus, V., Kinet, J.-M., 1999. NaCl effects on proline metabolismin rice (*Oryza sativa*) seedlings. *Physiologia Plantarum* 105 :450–458.

Maggio A., Reddy M.P., Joly R.J. (2000) Leaf gas exchange and solute accumulation in the halophyte Salvadora persica grown at moderate salinity. *Environ. Exp. Bot.* 44: 31-38.

Mansour M.M.F. (1998) Protection of plasma membrane of onion epidermal cells by glycine betaine and proline against NaCl stress. *Plant Physiol. Biochem.* 36: 767–772.

Misra N., Gupta A.K. (2005) Effect of salt stress on proline metabolism in two high yielding genotypes of green gram. *Plant Sci.* 169: 331–339.

Naidoo G., Kift J. (2006) Responses of the saltmarsh rush *Juncus kraussii* to salinity and water logging. *Aquatic Bot.* 84: 217-225.

Nedjimi B., Daoud Y., Touati M. (2006) Growth, water relations, proline and ion content of in vitro cultured *Atriplex halimus* subsp. *schweinfurthii* as affected by $CaCl_2$. *Communications in Biometry and Crop Science.* 1(2): 79–89.

Nedjimi B., Daoud Y. (2006) Effect of Na_2SO_4 on the growth, water relations, proline, total soluble sugars and ion content of *Atriplex halimus* subsp. schweinfurthii through in vitro culture. *Anal. Biol.* 28: 35–43.

Nedjimi B., Daoud Y., Touati M. (2007) Effet du stress salin sur la germination, la croissance et l'accumulalion ionique chez des jeunes plants d'*Atriplex halimus* subsp. *schweinfurthii* en culture *in vitro. Biotechnologie Végétale* 1 :49–55.

Nedjimi B., Daoud Y. (2009) Effects of calcium chloride on growth, membrane permeability and root hydraulic conductivity in two *Atriplex* species grown at high (sodium chloride) salinity. *Journal of Plant Nutrition* 32: 1818–1830.

Nedjimi B. (2011a) Rangeland improvement and management options in the arid steppes of Algeria. In: Germano M. Denise (eds) *Steppe ecosystems :*

Dynamics, land use and conservation, Nova Science Publishers, Inc : New York (in press).

Nedjimi, B., (2011b) Is salinity tolerance related to osmolytes accumulation in *Lygeum spartum* L. seedlings? Journal *of the Saudi Society of Agricultural Sciences* 10 (2), 80–87.

Nedjimi B. (2011c) *Résistance d'Atriplex halimus subsp. schweinfurthii aux sels solubles*. Éditions Universitaires Européennes, Sarrebruck, Allemagne, 204p.

Reddy A.R., Chaitanya K.V., Vivekanandan M. (2004) Drought-induced responses of photosynthesis and antioxidant metabolism in higher plants. *Journal of Plant Physiology* 161: 1189–1202.

Simiroff N., Cumbes Q.J. (1989) Hydroxyl radical scavenging activity of compatible solutes. *Phytochemistry* 28: 1057–1060.

Sivakumar P., Sharmila P., Parthasaradhi P. (2000) Proline alleviates salt stress induced enhancement in ribulose-1, 5-bisphosphate oxygenase activity. *Biochem. Biophys. Res. Commun.* 279: 512–515.

Song J., Feng G., Tian C., Zhang F. (2006b) Osmotic adjustment traits of *Suaeda physophora*, *Haloxylon ammodendron* and *Haloxylon persicum* in field or controlled conditions. *Plant Sci.* 170: 113–119.

Ueda A., Yamamoto-Yamane Y., Takabe T. (2007) Salt stress enhances proline utilization in the apical region of barley roots. *Bioch. Bioph. Research Comm.* 355: 61–66.

Veeranagamallaiah G., Chandraobulreddy P., Jyothsnakumari G., Sudhakar C. (2007) Glutamine synthetase expression and pyrroline-5-carboxylate reductase activity influence proline accumulation in two cultivars of foxtail millet (*Setaria italica* L.) with differential salt sensitivity. *Environ. Exp. Bot.* 60: 239-244.

Vicente O., Boscaiu M., Naranjo M.A., Estrelles E., Belles J.M., Soriano P. (2004) Responses to salt stress in the halophyte Plantago crassifolia (Plantaginaceae). *J. Arid Environ.* 58: 463-481.

Wang Z.Q., Yuan Y.Z., Ou J.Q., Lin Q.H., Zhang C.F. (2007) Glutamine synthetase and glutamate dehydrogenase contribute differentially to proline accumulation in leaves of wheat (*Triticum aestivum*) seedlings exposed to different salinity. *J. Plant Physiol.* 164: 695–701.

In: Proline
Editor: Bouzid Nedjimi
ISBN: 978-1-62257-739-2

Chapter II

Proline Cycle and Its Role in Secondary Metabolite Accumulation

María Perassolo, Ana María Giulietti and Julián Rodríguez Talou*
Microbiología Industrial y Biotecnología,
Facultad de Farmacia y Bioquímica, Universidad de Buenos Aires,
Buenos Aires, Argentina

Abstract

Proline is an amino acid that has been widely studied because of its multiple functions in plant cells. Accumulation of proline in response to different kinds of stress, such as drought, high salinity, UV irradiation and exposure to heavy metals is well documented. This amino acid has been described as exhibiting several functions in plant defense response, such as acting as a compatible osmolyte, having antioxidant properties and contributing to cell recovery after stress, among others.

Besides its central role in defense response, the influence of proline in secondary metabolite accumulation has been a subject of research. Shetty and

* Corresponding author: Julián Rodríguez Talou. E-mail: jrtalou@ffyb.uba.ar, jrodrigueztalou @yahoo.com.

co-workers have proposed that the proline cycle could be coupled to the pentose phosphate pathway (PPP), an important metabolic route that generates erithrose-4-phosphate. The latter compound is the precursor of the shikimate pathway, whose end-product (chorismate) becomes the branch point between primary and secondary metabolism and can lead to the synthesis of important secondary metabolites.

In the model proposed by Shetty, proline synthesis from glutamate generates two molecules of $NADP^+$, which act as cofactors of the first two enzymes in the PPP. Stimulating the proline cycle of biosynthesis and degradation could induce the PPP and generate an excess of erythrose-4-phosphate, thereby, driving the carbon flux towards the shikimate pathway.

In our work, we intend to review the effect of stimulating proline cycle on the accumulation of secondary metabolites, by the addition of proline analogs or precursors. Regarding this subject, we are going to discuss our findings related to anthraquinone production in *Rubia tinctorum* cell suspension cultures. Beside this, we will analyze the role of proline cycle in the defense response, focusing on its antioxidant activity and the effect on the final accumulation of secondary metabolites.

1. Introduction

Proline might be the most studied amino acid in nature. Many authors have reviewed its many functions in cell homeostasis. Not only is it essential in primary metabolism, but it is also involved in plant defense response to a variety of stresses [1]. In plant cells, the proline proportion in the pool of free amino acid increases from ~5% under normal conditions to 80% under stress conditions [2].

1.1. Biosynthesis of Proline and Proline Cycle

In plant cells, biosynthesis of proline is mainly achieved by pyrroline-5-carboxylate synthase (P5CS), which converts glutamate into P5C, and by P5C reductase (P5CR), which further transforms P5C into proline (see Figure 1) [1, 3]. As an alternative, P5C can be produced by transamination of ornithine, by ornithine-delta-aminotransferase (OAT) in the mitochondria, and can then be further converted into proline in the cytosol [1, 4]. Degradation, on the other hand, occurs in the mitochondria by the sequential action of proline dehydrogenase (PDH) and P5C dehydrogenase (P5CDH), generating P5C and glutamate, respectively [1, 3].

It is generally accepted that proline accumulation in response to stress is a consequence of an increase in its biosynthesis rather than a decrease in its degradation [3, 5], although there is evidence of a decrease in the rate of transcription and activity of PDH as a consequence of osmotic stress [4]. This particular amino acid has many advantages compared to others: it is the end product of a highly regulated pathway, it shows a limited involvement in transamination or decarboxylation reactions due to its chemical structure, and proves to be a very efficient way to store energy since its oxidation renders a high yield of ATP [6]. These and other facts make proline the preferred osmolyte to be accumulated during stress.

However, it should be noted that, besides its established role as osmolyte, proline accumulation during stress and its consequences are still under debate [4].

As it is discussed here later, stimulation of proline cycle and proline accumulation may be favorable to other processes, such as secondary metabolite accumulation.

1.2. The Pentose Phosphate Pathway and Its Role in Plant Homeostasis

As in all living organisms, glycolysis occurs in plant cells and is responsible for oxidation of sugars and the generation of pyruvate, as well as some ATP and NADH [7]. However, apart from glycolysis, plant cells have an alternative route for the oxidation of sugars: the pentose phosphate pathway (PPP). Located both in the cytosol and the plastids, this pathway begins with the oxidation of glucose-6-phosphate to render ribulose-5-phosphate CO_2 and reducing power that is kept as NADPH [7]. This is an essential role of the PPP, since this route becomes the main source of NADPH in non-photosynthetic cells, and under oxidative stress, is responsible for the maintenance of the redox potential [8]. Glucose-6-phosphate dehydrogenase (G6PDH) is the first enzyme in the pathway and, besides producing NADPH, is responsible for controlling the carbon flux through the PPP [9].

In the following steps of the PPP, ribulose-5-phosphate is converted by a series of reversible non-oxidative reactions into different sugars, which are precursors for the synthesis of different metabolites [8].

Not only does this route generate the precursors for the synthesis of nucleotides, but it also plays an essential role in secondary metabolite production, since it generates erythrose-4-phosphate, which is the substrate of the shikimate pathway [10]. The latter is responsible for the synthesis of aromatic amino acids and also is one of the main pathways involved in the biosynthesis of secondary metabolites, such as phenolics, flavonoids, lignin and anthraquinones.

Plant secondary metabolites have been extensively used as medicines in the pharmaceutical industry and are important constituents of aromatic plants used in the food industry.

Several of them are considered as nutraceuticals and their essential oils are the main compounds of many cosmetic products. Moreover, they play an important role in plant defense responses against pathogens.

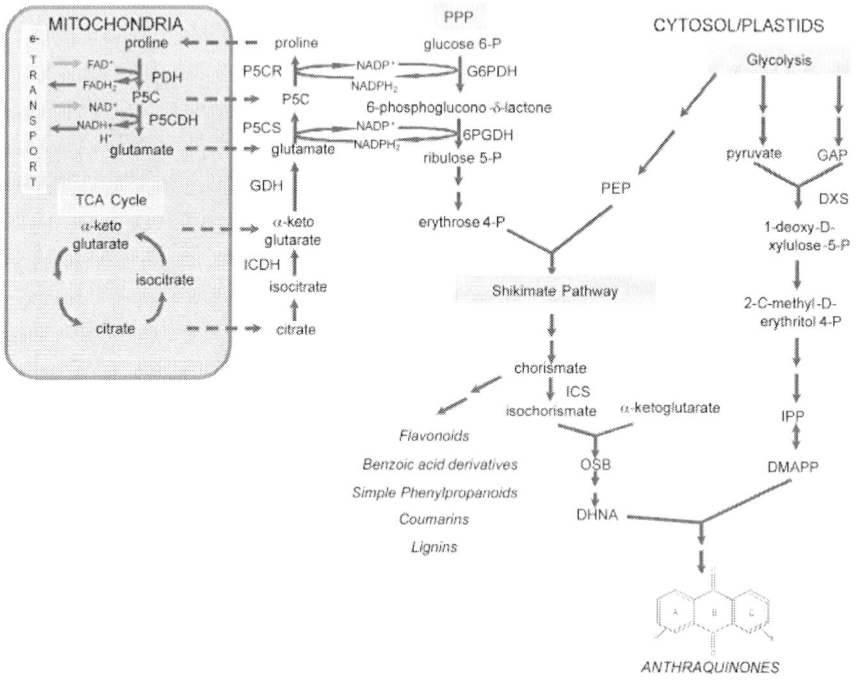

Figure 1. Schematic illustration of the metabolic pathways mentioned in this work. 6PGDH: 6-phosphogluconate dehydrogenase; DHNA: 1,4-dihydroxy-2-naphthoic acid; DMAPP: 3,3-dimethylallylpyrophosphate; DXS: 1-deoxy-D-xylulose 5-phosphate synthase; G6PDH: glucose-6-phosphate dehydrogenase; GAP: glyceraldehyde-3-phosphate; GDH: glutamate dehydrogenase; ICDH: isocitrate (NADP) dehydrogenase; ICS: isochorismate synthase; IPP: isopentenyl-5-pyrophosphate; OSB: *o*-succinylbenzoic acid; -P: phosphate; P5C: pyrroline-5-carboxylate; P5CDH: P5C dehydrogenase; P5CR: P5C reductase; P5CS: P5C synthetase; PDH: proline dehydrogenase PEP: phosphoenolpyruvate; PPP: pentose phosphate pathway; TCA: Tricarboxylic acids.

1.3. The Proline Linked-Pentose Phosphate Pathway

Shetty has proposed a model in which the proline cycle could be coupled to the first steps of the PPP [11]. In this model, the $NADP^+$ generated by the reduction of glutamate to proline could act as cofactor of the first enzymes in the PPP. Therefore, by modulating the proline cycle, it could be possible to increase the production of secondary metabolites.

Moreover, the excess of proline could replace NADH in oxidative phosphorylation inside the mitochondria [12].The proline-linked PPP has been described as being critical in providing erythrose-4-phosphate to shikimate and phenylpropanoid pathways.

Some authors have studied the P5C-Proline cycle. This cycle and its role in osmotic stress have been confirmed in model plants such as tobacco and arabidopsis by genetic engineering strategies [4]. In another work, it was observed that P5C-Proline cycle was also stimulated in arabidopsis by the pathogen *Pseudomonas syringae* [13]. It was also found that PDH and P5C reductase activities were increased in the presence of the avirulent strain. In addition to this, silenced-PDH plants showed reduced ROS levels and susceptibility to the avirulent strain, suggesting that PDH could be involved in hypersensitive response (HR) and disease resistance in Arabidopsis wild type plants. The authors proposed that activation of the P5C-Pro cycle could lower NADPH cytosolic levels, which are required for the activation of the PPP. However, in neither of these works was the relationship between the proline cycle, the PPP and secondary metabolism analyzed.

2. Biochemical Studies of the Proline Cycle, the PPP and Secondary Metabolite Accumulation

Modulation of the proline cycle can be achieved by the addition of precursors, such as proline or glutamate, and, also, of proline analogs, such as azetidine-2-carboxylic acid (A2C), and thiazolidine-4-carboxylic acid (T4C). It was demonstrated that T4C was a specific inhibitor of proline oxidation in barley mitochondria, since when it was added at 1 mM, it inhibited PDH but not the transport of proline through the inner mitochondria membrane [14].

The effect of A2C, another competitive inhibitor of PDH, on the synthesis of different phenolic compounds was extensively studied [12, 15-17]. In order to analyze the production of rosmarinic acid (RA, an hydroxycinnamic acid ester with antioxidant properties that is used as a food preservative) in shoot cultures of a clonal line of *Origanum vulgare*, Yang and Shetty evaluated different compounds: proline, its analog A2C, and two proline precursors, arginine and ornithine [12]. They found that proline content was increased in all the treatments performed (proline, arginine and ornithine, with or without A2C, and A2C alone) at 15 and 30 days of culture, and the same behavior was observed for RA production as well as total phenolics at 30 days. The cultures treated with A2C alone showed the lowest increase in proline content, but the production of RA at 15 days in these cultures was the highest. These results are consistent with the proposed model, since it was concluded that in the presence of A2C, both proline precursors were likely converted into proline in order to overcome A2C inhibition. Therefore proline synthesis and oxidation were enhanced, which resulted in increased RA and total phenolic content. Similar results were found by Lattanzio et al. (2009) when oregano plants were subjected to nutritional stress [15].

In another series of studies, proline (0.25 mM), A2C (200 μM) and a combination of both were used to evaluate their effect on the proline-linked PPP in germinating *Vicia fava* [16]. The three treatments resulted in an increase in total phenolics, L-DOPA and in proline accumulation, as well as stimulation of G6PDH activity. These results indicated that addition of A2C resulted in stimulation of proline-linked PPP, and, as a consequence, total phenolic production was enhanced. These phytochemicals are important for their antioxidant activity (phenolics), and L-DOPA has preventive action against Parkinson's disease.

As an interesting application of this model, tolerance to A2C was used as a complimentary screen to *Pseudomonas* tolerance for the selection of high phenolic producing clonal lines of *Lavandula angustifolia* Mill. [17]. Lavander is a plant used in food, medicine and cosmetic industry due to its essential oils and phenolic metabolites. This strategy arose from the fact that accumulation of phenolics is a common plant response to elicitation, and from the observation that in *Pseudomonas*-treated cultures, RA as well as proline content was increased.

We studied the role of the proline-linked PPP in the biosynthesis of anthraquinones (AQs). These secondary metabolites are produced by several plant species, including *Rubia tinctorum* and *Morinda citrifolia* [18]. Their carbon skeleton is derived by different metabolic pathways (see Figure 1): The A and B rings are originated from *o*-succinylbenzoate, which is formed by the condensation of α-ketoglutarate and isochorismate, whereas the isopentenyl pyrophosphate is the precursor of the C ring. Isochorismate is synthesized from chorismate, the end-product of the shikimate pathway, by the isochorismate synthase (ICS) [19]. Chorismate becomes the branch point in plant metabolism, since it is the precursor of several metabolic pathways, including those leading to aromatic amino acids, phenylpropanoids and flavonoids, among others.

AQs have been traditionally used as dyes in the textile industry and have a potential use in other industries due to their thermal and light stability. In addition to this, they have been described to exhibit interesting biological properties, including antifungal, antimicrobial, anticancer and antioxidant activities [10]. Recently, they have also been described as being useful in photodynamic therapy for the treatment of cancer [20]. These attributes make them interesting for studying their biosynthesis in plant in vitro cultures, as an attractive alternative for their production instead of the more environmentally harmful strategy of extracting them from their natural source. In addition to this, in vitro cultures have been widely used as a model in order to study different aspects of secondary metabolic pathways and their regulation [10].

Our study was focused on studying the role of the proline linked-PPP in the biosynthesis of AQs. Thus, we used different strategies with the aim of stimulating the proline cycle and evaluating the effects on the PPP and AQ production. We first evaluated the effect of proline on cell suspension cultures of *R. tinctorum* [21]. We found that the addition of 0.25 mM of proline resulted in an increase in the specific and volumetric content of AQs after the first 7 days of culture, and then it started to decrease until it reached control values. On the other hand, no induction of G6PDH was observed in these experiments. However, the carbon flux through the PPP was increased after the addition of proline, since biosynthesis of AQs was 50% higher.

In another set of experiments, we tested the effects of glutamate, which is the proline precursor in the proline cycle, on secondary metabolic pathways of *R. tinctorum* [10]. When added at 5 mM, glutamate enhanced AQ and total phenolics content (up to 30% and 12%, respectively, after 4 days of culture), as well as increased proline content (up to 130% after 2 days of culture). As before, no significant differences in G6PDH activity were observed between treatments. In order to further analyze the role of the proline linked-PPP, we treated *R. tinctorum* cell suspension cultures with two proline analogs: A2C (25 μM) and T4C (100 and 200 μM) [10]. All the treatments increased proline content after 7 days of culture (between 30% and 37%).The highest concentration of T4C impaired cell growth during the first days of culture, which was accompanied by a decrease in G6PDH activity at day 2 and a lesser production of AQs and total phenolics at day 4. However, at day 7, this treatment enhanced AQ content up to 27%, but no changes in G6PDH activity were observed.

The effects of the same proline analogs were tested in *M. citrifolia* cell suspension cultures [22]. Whereas the addition of 25 μM of A2C only increased proline accumulation after 6 days of culture (65%), the addition of 50 μM of A2C enhanced both proline and AQ content at day 6 (171% and 35%, respectively), but only proline content at day 10 (26%). The effects of T4C were only assayed at 100 μM, since a higher concentration (200 μM) severely impaired cell growth (as mentioned here before and in correlation with the observations of Tarmizi et al. [23]). Cells treated with T4C showed increases at both 6 and 10 days of culture, in AQ (40 and 36%, respectively) and proline content (117 and 51%, respectively). However, neither of the preformed treatments resulted in an increase in G6PDH activity, which correlates well with our previous results. It can be supposed that in spite of the increased demand of carbon skeletons from PPP, which are needed for the biosynthesis of AQs (and other secondary metabolites), the levels of G6PDH are not limiting the carbon flux through this pathway.

3. Studies of Proline Cycle, ROS, PPP and Secondary Metabolite Production in Plant Defense Responses

Production of ROS is an expected consequence of aerobic processes [2, 24], and therefore plant cells have developed different scavenging systems to detoxify them. However, under stress conditions, this antioxidant protection is overwhelmed and ROS content rises. An oxidative burst is a commonly observed event when plant cultures are treated with different elicitors, such as microbial preparations, wounding or plant-derived components [25]. These compounds are mainly produced by membrane-bound NADPH oxidase and, to a lesser extent, by apoplastic peroxidase [26]. Among their many actions, ROS are responsible for triggering hypersensitivity reactions and cell death, contributing to cell wall reinforcement, promoting gene activation and inducing the biosynthesis of defense compounds [25, 27]. Thus, the effects of ROS in the defense response can be classified into two distinct categories: they can cause severe damage and even plant death, but they also contribute with the plant defense response by inducing defense-related genes and by participating in signaling pathways [24].

As mentioned before, proline plays a central role in plant defense responses. Besides its well documented role as a compatible osmolyte, proline have been described to exhibit antioxidant activity, not only by reacting with ROS but also because it can stabilize and protect detoxifying enzymes [1]. Several authors have observed this protective activity of proline. Ozden et al. have reported that pretreatment of proline resulted in decreased production of H_2O_2 and lesser lipid peroxidation in leaves of *Vitis vinifera* L. subjected to H_2O_2 treatment [28]. In *Rosa hybrida* L., addition of 5 mM proline resulted in lower levels of $O_2^{\cdot -}$ and increased vase life [2]. This amino acid also contributes to cell recovery after stress by providing electrons to the respiratory chain and by acting as a nitrogen and carbon source [1, 5]. This proposed role of proline is in accordance with the rapid induction of PDH observed during stress recovery, as reviewed by Hare and Cress [3]. In addition to this, proline and its degradation products have been described to induce the expression of genes related to pathogen defense [29].

The role of ROS, signaling molecules in defense responses has also been studied in relation to proline biosynthesis. For instance, Skopelitis et al. observed that ROS generated by different kinds of stress induced the expression of the α-subunit of glutamate dehydrogenase (GDH) in tobacco and grapevine [30]. The exact role of this enzyme, which catalyzes both the amination and deamination of 2-oxoglutarate and glutamate, respectively, is not completely elucidated. In their work, the authors used different plant tissues of *N. tabacum* and *V. vinifera* var. Sultanina subjected to NaCl, ammonium or menadione stress. All of the treatments performed led to an increase in ROS content, in the transcription of the gene encoding the α-subunit of GDH and in a higher aminating GDH activity, among other effects. As a consequence, glutamate and proline content was increased. The authors propose that ROS are a signal involved in the induction of GDH, in addition or as an alternative to hyperammonia.

Other works also studied the role of GDH in proline accumulation during stress. Wang et al. analyzed the role of glutamine synthetase (GS) and GDH in glutamate production under salinity stress in *Triticum aestivum* [5]. They observed that under high salinity conditions (300 mM NaCl), the increase in proline accumulation was accompanied by an increase in glutamate content and GDH activity, whereas GS activity was decreased.

As it was outlined before, the PPP is essential in plant cell metabolism and physiology since it provides NADPH and carbon skeletons for the synthesis of secondary metabolites. Therefore, since a defense response has an increased demand of both reducing power and carbon precursors [31], the PPP plays an important role in plant defenses. Moreover, G6PDH activity was described to be essential in human erythrocytes to overcome oxidative stress, since this enzyme was the only source of NADPH [9].

The importance of the PPP in defense responses is analyzed by several authors. For instance, Wang et al. studied the role of glucose-6-phosphate dehydrogenase (G6PDH), the key enzyme in the PPP, in modulating the levels of reduced glutathione (GSH) in callus culture of two ecotypes of *Phragmites communis* Trin. [9]. Since it belongs to the antioxidant defense, two molecules of GSH are oxidized to render glutathione disulfide (GSSG). Regeneration of GSH is accomplished by the action of glutathione redutase (GR) with NADPH as a cofactor. These authors found that a decrease in both G6PDH activity and expression was accompanied by a decrease in GR activity, GSH levels and, also, in glutathione peroxidase activity (GPX, an enzyme involved in H_2O_2 detoxification by GSH). They also observed that H_2O_2 was responsible for inducing GR, GPX and G6PDH activities and also for increasing GSH levels.

The advantages of higher G6PDH activity and consequently increased NADPH levels were studied by Scharte et al. [31]. They infiltrated resistant and susceptible tobacco cultivars with zoospores of *Phytophthora nicotianae* and they observed an almost 3-fold increase in G6PDH activity in the resistant cultivar, whereas the susceptible one had a slower and smaller increase (only 25%). Experiments performed with glucosamine-6-phosphate, an inhibitor of G6PDH, confirmed the essential role of this enzyme in the defense response. Given the fact that one of the two plastidic isoforms of the G6PDH is less sensitive to rising NADPH levels than the cytosolic one, the authors expressed a plastidic P2 isoform from *Arabidopsis* in the cytosol of the susceptible tobacco cultivars. The transgenic lines obtained showed improved tolerance to infection with *P. nicotianae* when compared to wild type cultivars. Moreover, these transgenic lines showed enhanced drought tolerance and flowering, which has potential applications in agronomic traits.

In order to study the proline-linked PPP in defense responses, we performed an assay with Methyl jasmonate (MeJ), a well-known endogenous elicitor that has been widely used to enhance secondary metabolite production. Our goal was to analyze the role of ROS, proline cycle and PPP in *R. tinctorum* cell suspension cultures after MeJ elicitation [27]. We found that elicitation with MeJ resulted in an increase in both proline and AQ content, whereas treatment with diphenyliodonium (DPI, an inhibitor of NADPH oxidase which is the main source of ROS) abolished these effects. Treatment with both glucose and glucose oxidase (a H_2O_2-generating system), mimicked the effects of MeJ, indicating that H_2O_2 was a signal involved in both processes. Again, all the treatments performed failed to induce PPP, since no changes in G6PDH activity were observed. Therefore, these findings are in accordance with the hypothesis we have previously outlined.

In these experiments, we also evaluated the activity of both GDH (involved in glutamate production from α-ketoglutarate in the aminating reaction, as we mentioned earlier) and isocitrate (NADP) dehydrogenase (ICDH, an enzyme involved in the synthesis of α-ketoglutarate). While the activity of ICDH remained unchanged, GDH activity showed a drastic increase after MeJ elicitation (between 100% and 171%). These changes in GDH activity are similar to those reported by Skopelitis et al. [30] and Wang et al. [5]. It can be assumed that, as commented before, ROS enhances proline accumulation by increasing GDH activity in *R. tintorum*.

Conclusion

Proline is an amino acid that contributes to plant cell homeostasis in a variety of ways. There is some evidence that stimulating the proline cycle with analogs or precursors results in an increase in proline content and a higher carbon flux through the PPP and, therefore, a higher production of secondary metabolites. The effect of ROS as a signal involved in the induction of proline accumulation and secondary metabolite production is also discussed. Although a complete understanding of proline functions is still missing, it is absolutely clear that its role in plant physiology is not limited to being just a precursor of protein biosynthesis and osmolyte.

In the present work, we have discussed some aspects of the regulation of proline biosynthesis and its involvement in secondary metabolite accumulation in plants. In many plant species, the essential role of proline-linked PPP and its effect on the biosynthesis of secondary metabolites was demonstrated, especially for those metabolites produced by the phenylpropanoid pathway.

In *R. tinctorum* and *M. citrifolia* in vitro cultures, it was shown that the stimulation of the proline cycle, which resulted in higher intracellular levels of proline, was correlated with an increase in AQ production. This correlation was observed after the addition of proline analogs and also in response to MeJ elicitation. However, no induction of G6PDH, which is the key enzyme in the PPP, was observed; therefore, this route would not be a limiting factor for providing the shikimate pathway with carbon skeletons for the biosynthesis of secondary metabolites.

The essential role of proline cycle in osmotic and saline stresses, as well as in defense against pathogens, has been demonstrated by genetic engineering in model plants, such as arabidopsis or tobacco. Although the effect on the PPP and secondary metabolite accumulation was not analyzed, it should be noticed that the more important factor in the defense response against biotic and abiotic stresses would be the continuous cycle of biosynthesis and degradation, rather than the accumulation of proline. Not only would this cycle produce higher levels of proline (antioxidant and stabilizer of macromolecules), but it also would help to maintain the redox balance in plant cells under stress.

The application of metabolic strategies on these biosynthetic pathways turned out to be successful in order to improve plant resistance to osmotic and saline stresses. These results are promising for the application of these strategies for increasing secondary metabolite accumulation in economically valuable plants, not only for the pharmaceutical industry but also for agricultural purposes.

Acknowledgments

This work was supported by grant PICT 14-15112 and 14-33166, ANPCyT (Agencia Nacional de Promoción Científica y Tecnológica), Argentina, and by grant UBACyT B181, Universidad de Buenos Aires. P.M., R.T.J. and G.A.M. are researchers from CONICET (Consejo Nacional de Investigaciones Científicas y Técnicas), Argentina.

References

[1] Szabados, L., Savoure, A. Proline: a multifunctional amino acid. *Trends Plant Sci.* 2010;15:89-97.

[2] Kumar,N., Pal, M., Singh, A., SaiRam, R. K., Srivastava, G. C. Exogenous proline alleviates oxidative stress and increase vase life in rose (*Rosa hybrida* L. 'Grand Gala'). *Scientia Horticulturae* 2010;127:79-85.

[3] Hare, P. D., Cress, W., van Staden, J. Proline synthesis and degradation: a model system for elucidating stress related signal transduction. *Journal of Experimental Botany* 1999;50:413-434.

[4] Miller, G., Honig, A., Stein, H., Suzuki, N., Mittler, R., Zilberstein, A. Unraveling delta1-pyrroline-5-carboxylate-proline cycle in plants by uncoupled expression of proline oxidation enzymes. *J. Biol. Chem.* 2009;284:26482-26492.

[5] Wang, Z. Q., Yuan, Y. Z., Ou, J. Q., Lin, Q. H., Zhang, C. F. Glutamine synthetase and glutamate dehydrogenase contribute differentially to proline accumulation in leaves of wheat (*Triticum aestivum*) seedlings exposed to different salinity. *J. Plant Physiol.* 2007;164:695-701.

[6] Hare, P. D., Cress, W. A. Metabolic implications of stress-induced proline accumulation in plants. *Plant Growth Regulation* 1997;21:79-102.

[7] Taiz, L., Zieger, E. *Plant Physiology*. Sinauer; 2002.

[8] Kruger, N. J., von Schaewen, A. The oxidative pentose phosphate pathway: structure and organisation. *Curr. Opin. Plant Biol.* 2003;6:236-246.

[9] Wang, X., Ma, Y., Huang, C., Wan, Q., Li, N., Bi, Y. Glucose-6-phosphate dehydrogenase plays a central role in modulating reduced glutathione levels in reed callus under salt stress. *Planta* 2008;227:611-623.

[10] Perassolo, M., Quevedo, C. V., Giulietti, A. M., Rodríguez Talou, J. Stimulation of the proline cycle and anthraquinone accumulation in *Rubia tinctorum* cell suspension cultures in the presence of glutamate and two proline analogs. *Plant Cell Tiss. Organ. Cult.* 2011;106:153–159.

[11] Shetty, K. Role of proline-linked pentose phosphate pathway in biosynthesis of plant phenolics for functional food and environmental applications: a review. *Process Biochem.* 2004;39:789–803.

[12] Yang, R., Shetty, K. Stimulation of Rosmarinic Acid in Shoot Cultures of Oregano (*Origanum vulgare*) Clonal Line in Response to Proline, Proline Analogue, and Proline Precursors. *J. Agric. Food Chem.* 1998;46:2888-2893.

[13] Cecchini, N. M., Monteoliva, M. I., Alvarez, M. E. Proline dehydrogenase contributes to pathogen defense in Arabidopsis. *Plant Physiol.* 2011;155:1947-1959.

[14] Elthon, T. E., Stewart, C. R. Effects of the Proline Analog L-Thiazolidine-4-carboxylic Acid on Proline Metabolism. *Plant Physiol.* 1984;74:213-218.

[15] Lattanzio, V., Cardinali, A., Ruta, C., Fortunato, I. M., Lattanzio, V. M. T., Linsalata, V., Cicco, N. Relationship of secondary metabolism to growth in oregano (Origanum vulgare L.) shoot cultures under nutritional stress. *Environmental and Experimental Botany* 2009;65:54-62.

[16] Shetty, P., Atallah, M. T., Shetty, K. Stimulation of total phenolics, L-DOPA and antioxidant activity through proline-linked pentose phosphate pathway in response to proline and its analogue in germinating fava beans (*Vicia faba*). *Process Biochem.* 2003;38:1707-1717.

[17] Al-Amier, H., Mansour, B. M., Toaima, N., Korus, R. A., Shetty, K. Tissue culture based screening for selection of high biomass and phenolic producing clonal lines of lavender using pseudomonas and azetidine-2-carboxylate. *J. Agric. Food Chem.* 1999;47:2937-2943.

[18] Han, Y. S., Van der Heijden, R., Verpoorte, R. Biosynthesis of anthraquinones in cell cultures of the Rubiaceae. *Plant Cell Tiss. Organ Cult.* 2001;67:201-220.

[19] Quevedo, C., Perassolo, M., Alechine, E., Corach, D., Giulietti, A. M., Talou, J. R. Increasing anthraquinone production by overexpression of 1-

deoxy-D-xylulose-5-phosphate synthase in transgenic cell suspension cultures of *Morinda citrifolia*. *Biotechnol. Lett.* 2010;32:997-1003.

[20] Comini, L. R., Fernandez, I. M., Rumie Vittar, N. B., Nunez Montoya, S. C., Cabrera, J. L., Rivarola, V. A. Photodynamic activity of anthraquinones isolated from *Heterophyllaea pustulata* Hook f. (Rubiaceae) on MCF-7c3 breast cancer cells. *Phytomedicine* 2011;18:1093-1095.

[21] Perassolo, M., Quevedo, C., Busto, V., Ianone, F., Giulietti, A. M., Rodríguez Talou, J. Enhance of anthraquinone production by effect of proline and aminoindan-2-phosphonic acid in *Rubia tinctorum* suspension cultures. *Enzyme and Microbial Technology* 2007;41:181-185.

[22] Quevedo, C. V., Perassolo, M., Giulietti, A. M., Talou, J. R. Enhancement of anthraquinone production in *Morinda citrifolia* cell suspension cultures after stimulation of the proline cycle with two proline analogs. *Biotechnol. Lett.* 2011.

[23] Tarmizi, A. H., Marziah, M. Studies towards understanding proline accumulation in oil plam (*Elaeis guineensis* Jacq.) polyembryogenic cultures. *J. Oil Palm. Res.* 2000;12:8-13.

[24] Apel, K., Hirt, H. Reactive oxygen species: metabolism, oxidative stress, and signal transduction. *Annu. Rev. Plant Biol.* 2004;55:373-399.

[25] Orozco-Cardenas, M. L., Narvaez-Vasquez, J., Ryan, C. A. Hydrogen peroxide acts as a second messenger for the induction of defense genes in tomato plants in response to wounding, systemin, and methyl jasmonate. *Plant Cell* 2001;13:179-191.

[26] Zhao, J., Davis, L. C., Verpoorte, R. Elicitor signal transduction leading to production of plant secondary metabolites. *Biotechnol. Adv.* 2005;23:283-333.

[27] Perassolo, M., Quevedo, C. V., Busto, V. D., Giulietti, A. M., Talou, J. R. Role of reactive oxygen species and proline cycle in anthraquinone accumulation in *Rubia tinctorum* cell suspension cultures subjected to methyl jasmonate elicitation. *Plant Physiol. Biochem.* 2011;49:758-763.

[28] Ozden, M., Demirel, U., Kahraman, A. Effects of proline on antioxidant system in leaves of grapevine (*Vitis vinifera* L.) exposed to oxidative stress by H_2O_2. *Scientia Horticulturae* 2009;119:163-168.

[29] Deuschle, K., Funck, D., Forlani, G., Stransky, H., Biehl, A., Leister, D., van der Graaff, E., Kunze, R., Frommer, W. B. The role of $[D]^1$-pyrroline-5-carboxylate dehydrogenase in proline degradation. *Plant Cell* 2004;16:3413-3425.

[30] Skopelitis, D. S., Paranychianakis, N. V., Paschalidis, K. A., Pliakonis, E. D., Delis, I. D., Yakoumakis, D. I., Kouvarakis, A., Papadakis, A. K., Stephanou, E. G., Roubelakis-Angelakis, K. A. Abiotic stress generates ROS that signal expression of anionic glutamate dehydrogenases to form glutamate for proline synthesis in tobacco and grapevine. *Plant Cell* 2006;18:2767-2781.

[31] Scharte, J., Schon, H., Tjaden, Z., Weis, E., von Schaewen, A. Isoenzyme replacement of glucose-6-phosphate dehydrogenase in the cytosol improves stress tolerance in plants. *Proc. Natl. Acad. Sci. US* 2009;106:8061-8066.

In: Proline
Editor: Bouzid Nedjimi

ISBN: 978-1-62257-739-2

Chapter III

Small Organic Molecules Based on the L-Proline for Catalyzing the Asymmetric Reaction

***Lingyan Liu*[*], *Bin Wang, Weixing Chang and Jing Li*[*†]**
State Key Laboratory of Elemento-Organic Chemistry, The College of Chemistry, Nankai University, Tianjin, People's Republic of China

Abstract

A few new prolinethioamide compounds, designed and prepared from readily available natural amino acid L-proline and L-valine, have been found to be active catalysts for the direct aldol reaction of various aldehydes with acetone, cyclohexanone or cyclopentanone at 0°C or rt. Using only 2 mol% or 0.2 mol% loading of organocatalysts 1 or 2, the reaction could give high enantioselectivity with up to 96% enantiomeric excess for the reaction of 2-nitrobenzaldehyde with acetone or higher than 99% ee for the reaction of 3-nitrobenzaldehyde with acetone in aqueous media, respectively. Moreover, using the simple dipeptide derivative 3, we unexpectedly found the different regioselectivity product, 1,2-diol and 1,4-diol, could be achieved with high

[*] State Key Laboratory of Elemento-Organic Chemistry, the college of Chemistry, Nankai University, Tianjin 300071, People's Republic of China, E-mail: liulingyan@nankai.edu.cn.
[†*] State Key Laboratory of Elemento-Organic Chemistry, the college of Chemistry, Nankai University, Tianjin 300071, People's Republic of China, E-mail: lijing@nankai.edu.cn.

yields and high enantioselectivities in the reaction of hydroxyl acetone and aromatic aldehydes promoted by the different additives at room temperature. Summarily, these structurally simple catalysts have been proven to be highly efficient prolinethioamide derivatives in asymmetric aldol reaction. In addition, we also explored a few known organocatalysts derived from L-proline application for some organic reaction. For example, the L-proline 4 has been found that it can catalyze well the ring-opening of epoxide with allylmetal reagent. And the catalyst 5 could promote the asymmetric allylation of aldehyde. The N-oxide compound 6 could effectively catalyze the ring-opening of epoxide and halide atom donor. The organophophine compound 7 is a highly efficient catalyst in the asymmetric Michael reaction of chalcone and cyclohexanone in our work (Figure 1). Our further work would mainly focus on the design and synthesis of polymer-supported L-proline or L-proline derivatives with tunable morphology. And the relationship between the structure and catalytic activity of these catalysts would also be investigated.

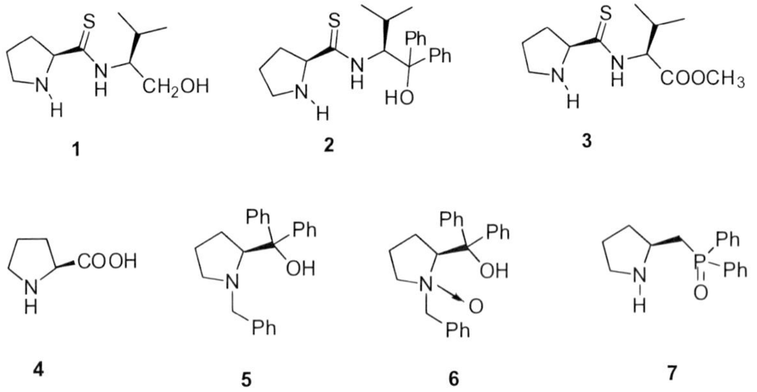

Figure 1. Several organocatalysts derived from L-proline.

The asymmetric catalysis is currently one of the most active areas of chemical development. It provides a strong theoretical foundation and academic basis for the exploration of chiral drugs, materials and spices. It is well known that the enzymes and metal complexes are two types of the most important and most effective catalysts. Especially, the metal complexes have been widely used to catalyze various asymmetric transformations and thus made important achievement, some of them have been applied to industrial production. Moreover, the 2001 Nobel Prize in Chemistry has been awarded to the three scientists who have made outstanding contributions in the field of asymmetric reaction catalyzed by metal complexes. In 1970, Hajos and Wiechert research groups firstly reported that the intramolecular aldol reaction could smoothly proceed in the presence of natural amino acid L-proline and obtain high enantioselective products (Scheme 1) [1].

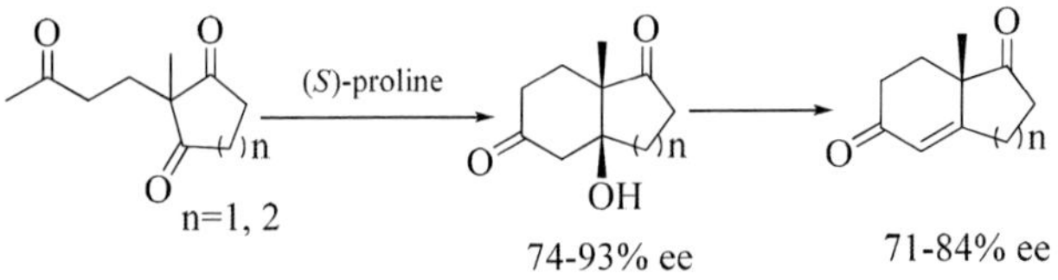

Scheme 1. The intramolecular aldol reaction.

In the following long period of time, the organocatalysis has not attracted the peoples' attention. Until 2000, the List research group reported the L-proline could also efficiently catalyze the intermolecular aldol reaction and afford high enantioselective products (**Scheme 2**) [2].

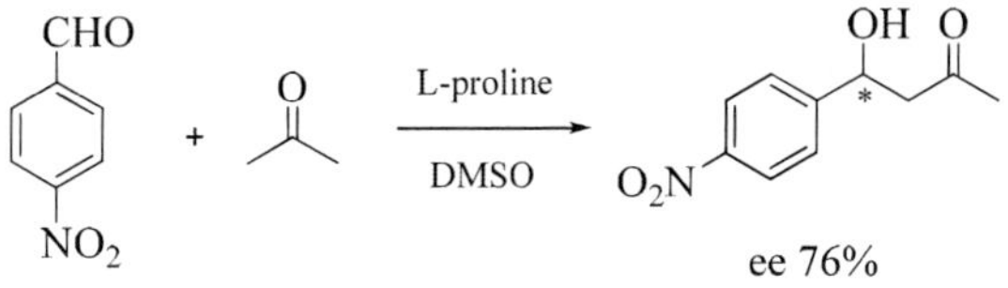

Scheme 2. The direct asymmetric aldol reation of acetone and aldehyde.

This report again ignites the chemists' interests on the research of organocatalysis. And then, the organocatalysis, in which small organic molecules (organo-catalysts) act as catalytically active species, has grown explosively to become one of the most exciting research areas in current organic chemistry [3]. One of the main advantages of organocatalysis is that organocatalysts can promote various organic transformations through unique activation patterns [4] compared to transition metal catalysis. In addition, the organocatalysis has the advantages of operationally simple and reaction green. For example, 1) no metal is needed to intrigue the reaction and do not worry about the toxic metal released into the environment; 2) the organic catalysts are usually inexpensive, easy to modify and prepare; 3) the organocatalysis reaction usually proceed in the air and do not need control the harsh anhydrous anaerobic conditions; 4) the organic catalysts is easily separated from products and may be recycled for several times, such as L-proline is soluble in water, insoluble in organic solvents.

L-proline, inexpensive and easily available, acting as the small organic molecule catalyst, has been widely used in the asymmetric aldol reaction and other asymmetric reactions, such as the Mannich reaction, Michael reaction, and so on. And great successes have been achieved. It is ascribed to proline itself characteristics which are as follows: 1) proline is a bifunctional groups compound in the catalytic reaction. It can be used as either a Lewis acid or a

Lewis base, similar to the enzyme catalysis; 2) the pyrolidine ring is favor to form the imine ion or stable enamine intermediate, and the rigid five-membered ring structure is conducive for the enantioselectivity induction. However, there are still some shortcomings about the proline. For instance, the usually long reaction time, the great amount of catalyst loading, or the strong polar solvent such as DMSO used because of its insolubility in many other solvents.

Due to these drawbacks, the chemists began to design and synthesize other more highly efficient small organic molecule catalysts based on the proline special structure.

1. The Profiles of Small Organic Molecules Catalysis Based on the L-Proline

With the rapid development of asymmetric reaction research, more and more novel small organic molecules catalysts derived from proline are designed, synthesized and applied in the asymmetric reaction. Such as the peptides, amino alcohols, diamines and tetra-azole acids, etc.

In 2003, Gong research group firstly reported that the asymmetric aldol reaction of acetone and aldehydes was catalyzed by the prolinamide with the multifunctional groups and resulted in the hydroxy ketone products with high yields and high enantioselectivities (Scheme 3) [5].

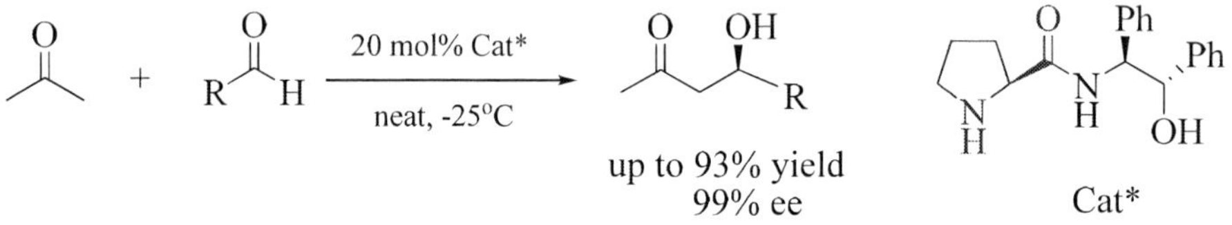

Scheme 3. The asymmetric aldol reaction of acetone and aldehydes catalyzed by the L-prolinamide.

From then on, it broke the traditional view in which the carboxyl group of amino acid is essential and prolinamide could not catalyze the aldol reaction. More and more novel structural prolinamide organocatalysts are successively prepared and applied in the asymmetric aldol reaction (Figure 2) [6].

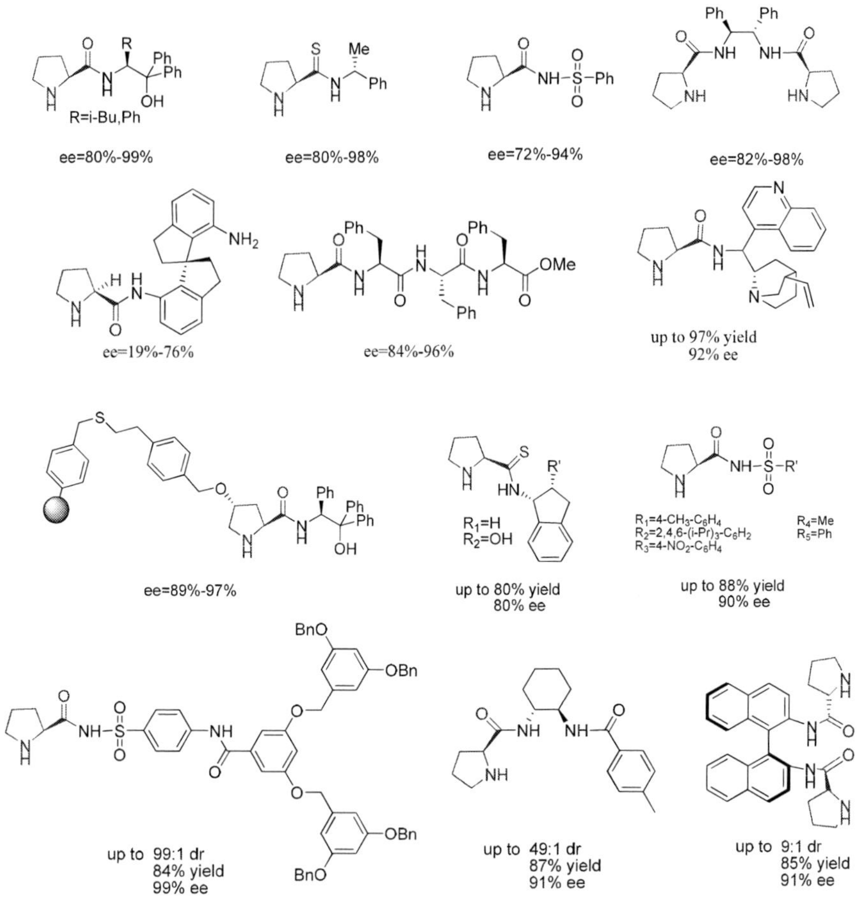

Figure 2. various prolinamide catalysts used in the asymmetric aldol reaction.

Although there are great amount of successful reports on the small organic molecules catalyzing the asymmetric aldol reaction, we found that the amount of catalyst loading was still larger and usually need about 10 mol% or more than 10 mol%. In comparison, there are few literatures reported about using less than 10 mol% catalyst loading or even less than 1 mol%. Hence, it is still the hot issue of research for the chemists to seek a more efficient catalyst system and further reduce the amount of catalyst. Additionally, the reported asymmetric aldol reactions are usually performed in the organic solvents or largely excessive acetone, the aqueous media asymmetric aldol reaction research has become the main trend with the rapid development of green chemistry and remains a challenge.

2. Our Research Work on the Small Organic Molecules Catalysts of L-Proline

Based on the above facts, our research group began to focus on the small organic molecules catalysis asymmetric reactions. Namely, by continuously modification and transformation of the proline structure, we engaged into designing and synthesizing more novel and simple prolinamide directly derived from natural amino acids proline and valine.

In our work, a few new prolinethioamide catalysts, designed and prepared from readily available natural amino acid L-proline and amino acid L-valine (Figure 3), have been found to be active catalysts for the direct aldol reaction of various aldehydes with acetone, cyclohexanone or cyclopentanone at 0°C or rt.

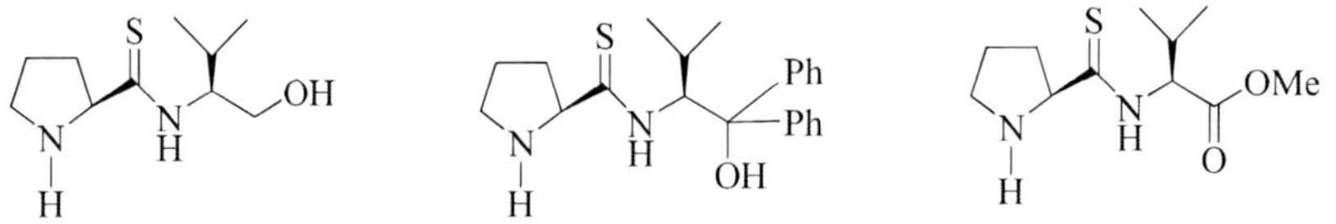

1 **2** **3**

Figure 3. The organocatalysts of L-prolinethioamide.

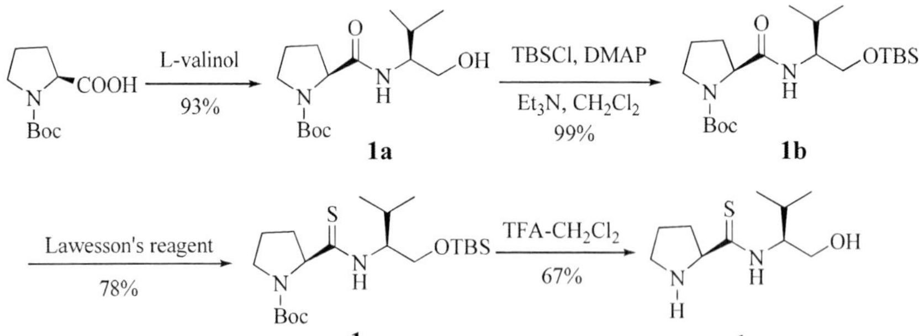

Scheme 4. Synthesis of prolinethioamide derivative **1**.

Using only 2 mol% or 0.2 mol% loading of organocatalysts 1 or 2, the reaction could give high enantioselectivity with up to 96% enantiomeric excess for the reaction of 2-nitrobenzaldehyde with acetone or higher than 99% ee for the reaction of 3-nitrobenzaldehyde with acetone in aqueous media, respectively.

Moreover, using the simple dipeptide derivative 3, we unexpectedly found the different regioselectivity product, 1,2-diol and 1,4-diol, could be achieved with high yields and high enantioselectivities in the reaction of between hydroxyl acetone and aromatic aldehydes promoted by the different additives at room temperature. Summarily, these structurally simple catalysts have been proven to be highly efficient prolinethioamide derivatives in asymmetric aldol reaction.

2.1. The Synthesis of Chiral Catalysts 1-3

The organocatalysts 1-3 were prepared from N-Boc-L-proline, reacted with the appropriate L-valinol or L-valinate, followed by the general strategy involving the protection of hydroxyl group with TBSCl, thiation with Lawesson's reagent and deprotection of the amino and hydroxyl functions under standard conditions (Scheme 4 and 5) [7].

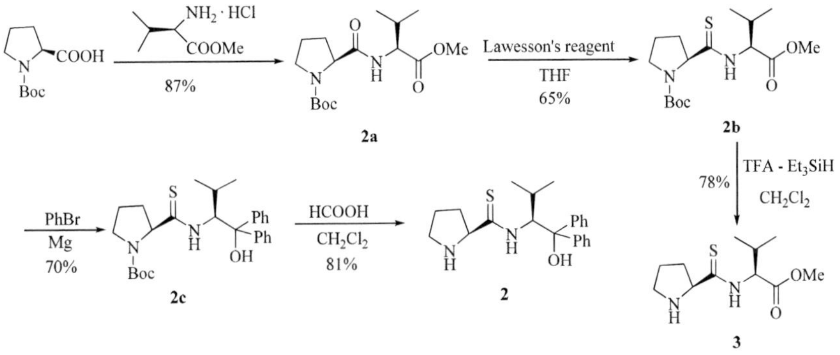

Scheme 5. Synthesis of prolinethioamide derivatives **2** and **3**.

2.2. The Application of Chiral Catalysts 1-3 in the Asymmetric Aldol Reaction of Aldehydes and Ketones

After synthesizing the above several new prolinethioamide catalysts, we attempt to use them in the direct asymmetric aldol reaction of aldehydes and acetone. This reaction is an important method to form carbon-carbon bond which provides straightforward access to the optically active β-hydroxycarbonyl structural unit found in many natural products and drugs [8]. Of course, all reaction parameters (including catalyst and its loading, temperature, solvent and additive, etc.) are the key research points, because any one of them may affect the reaction efficiency. Thus, we step by step examined these reaction conditions. As a result, we found that the simple prolinethioamide catalyst 1, prepared from L-proline and L-valinol, could efficiently promote the direct asymmetric aldol reaction of acetone and various aromatic aldehydes. Using only 2 mol% this catalyst loading, the reaction could smoothly proceed at zero or room temperature and afford the corresponding hydroxyl ketone products with high up to 96% enantioselectivity (Figure 4). It's important to mention that the terminal hydroxyl group of the organocatalyst 1 is a primary alcohol which is different from previously reported pre-requisited secondary or tertiary alcohol. The present studies have demonstrated the key role of combination of privileged chiral backbone and hydrogen bonding interactions in the asymmetric aldol reaction.

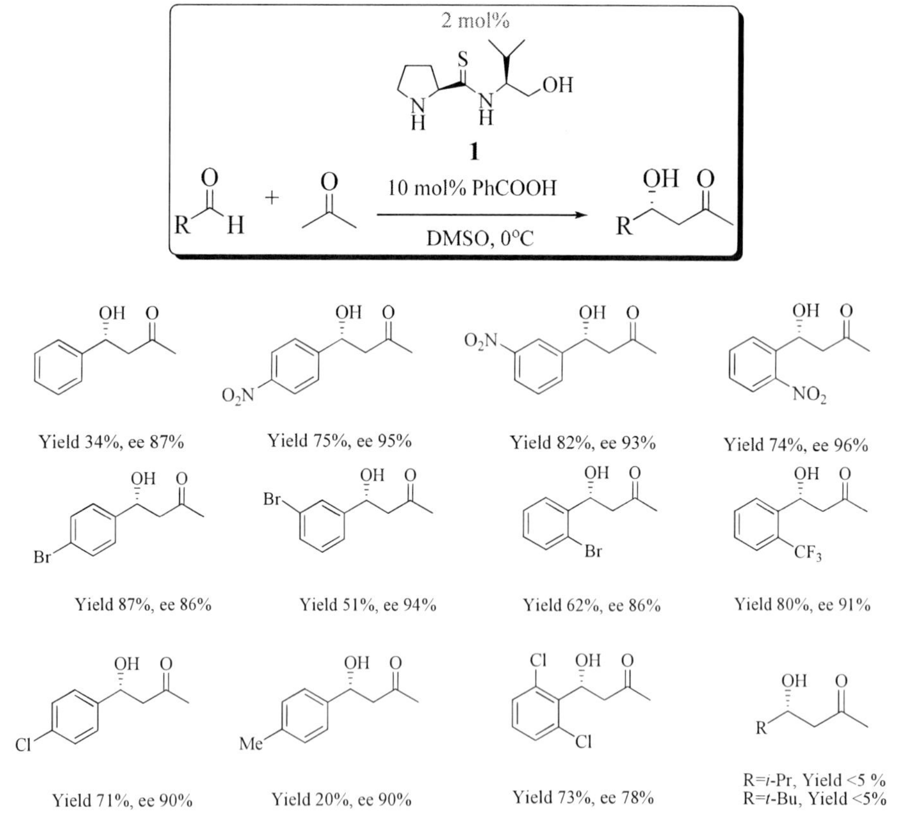

Figure 4. The corresponding aldol products.

Except for the acetone, the cyclohexanone could also act as donor to carry out the asymmetric aldol reaction in the presence of the prolinethioamide catalysts 1. Moreover, this reaction was carried out in pure water, thus this is 'green' to some degree. Reaction of cyclohexanone with a variety of electron-deficient aromatic aldehydes containing a variety of substitution patterns provided the desired *anti*-aldol products in high isolated yields (83-95%) with excellent diastereo- (95/5 to 99/1 dr) and enantioselectivities (96-99% ee) (Figure 5). Whereas the reaction could not proceed smoothly with non-activated aldehydes, such as benzaldehyde, 4-methylbenzaldehyde, and 4-methoxybenzaldehyde even prolonging the reaction time and only to give the aldol adducts in low yields but high enantioselectivities, respectively. In the case of cyclopentanone, the reaction could also give the product with high yield and excellent enantioselectivity but low diastereo-selectivity.

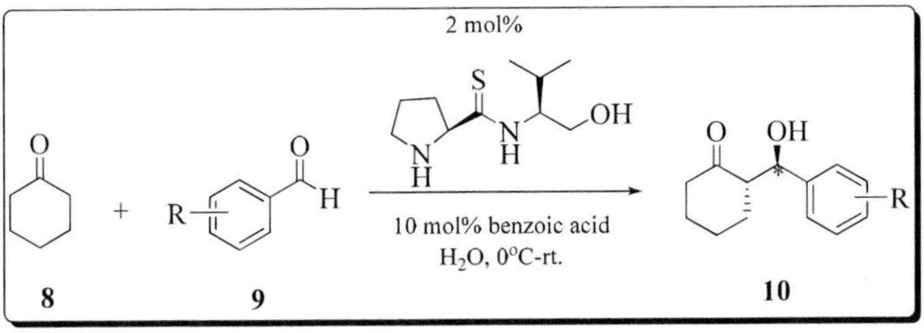

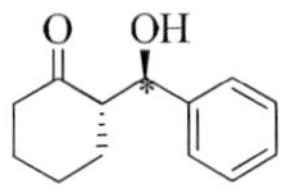

Yield 46%, ee 96% (*anti*)
anti:syn=95:5

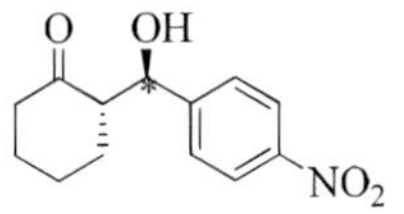

Yield 92%, ee 96% (*anti*)
anti:syn=99:1

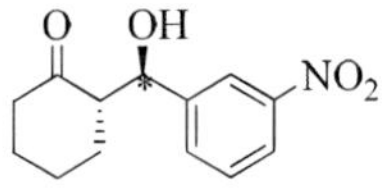

Yield 95%, ee 99% (*anti*)
anti:syn=96:4

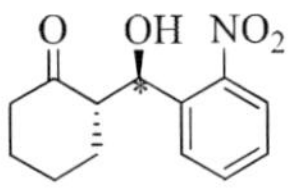

Yield 94%, ee 97% (*anti*)
anti:syn=98:2

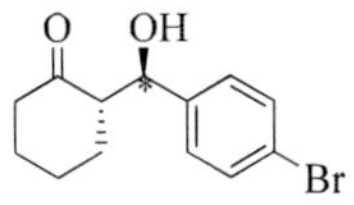

Yield 91%, ee 97% (*anti*)
anti:syn=97:3

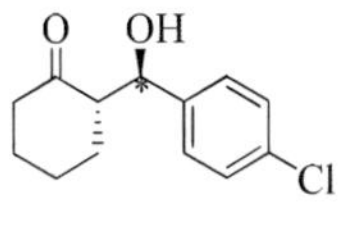

Yield 83%, ee 96% (*anti*)
anti:syn=95:5

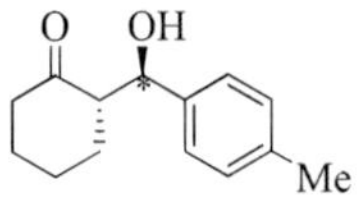

Yield 42%, ee 94% (*anti*)
anti:syn=97:3

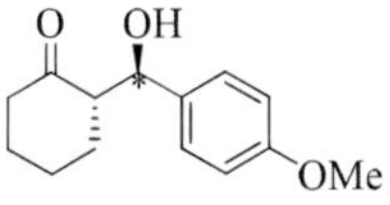

Yield 36%, ee 92% (*anti*)
anti:syn=97:3

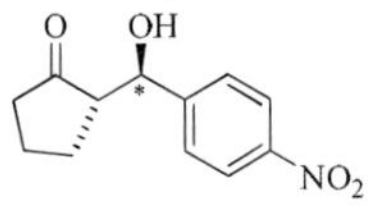

Yield 88%, ee 98% (*anti*)
anti:syn=67:33

Figure 5. The corresponding aldol products.

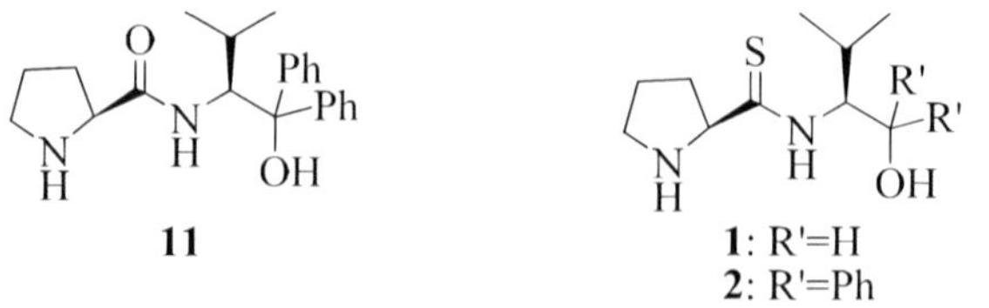

Figure 6. The prolinamide catalyst and the prolinethioamide catalyst.

Table 1. The direct asymmetric aldol reactions of acetone with various aldehydes catalyzed by organocatalyst 2 in aqueous media [a]

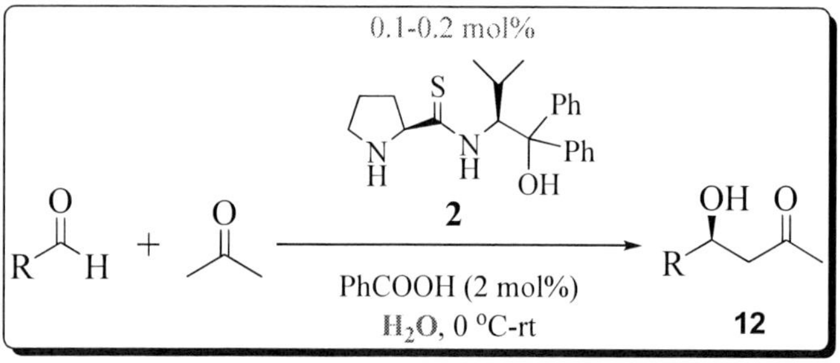

Entry	R	Product	Time (h)	Yield (%)[b]	ee (%)[c]
1	Ph	**12a**	16	92	97
2	4-$NO_2C_6H_4$	**12b**	12	92	95
3 [d]	3-$NO_2C_6H_4$	**12c**	12	88	>99
4 [d]	2-$NO_2C_6H_4$	**12d**	12	98	99
5	4-BrC_6H_4	**12e**	16	76	96
6	3-BrC_6H_4	**12f**	16	91	>99
7	2-BrC_6H_4	**12g**	16	90	98
8 [d]	4-$CF_3C_6H_4$	**12h**	10	91	98
9 [d]	2-$CF_3C_6H_4$	**12i**	10	96	99
10	4-FC_6H_4	**12j**	16	89	98
11	4-ClC_6H_4	**12k**	16	90	98
12	4-MeC_6H_4	**12l**	24	72	98
13	β-naphthyl	**12m**	12	77	96
14	2-Furyl	**12n**	12	67	84
15	*i*-Pr	**12o**	36	<10	-

[a] Unless stated otherwise, the reaction was carried out with acetone (0.2 mL, 2.5 mmol, 5 equiv.) and various aldehyde (0.5 mmol, 1 equiv.) under optimal reaction conditions in the presence of 0.2 mol% organocatalyst **2**. [b] Isolated yield. [c] Determined by chiral HPLC analysis using Chiralpak AD-H, AS-H or OJ-H column, and the configuration was assigned as *R* by comparison of optical rotation. [d] The reaction was carried out in the presence of 0.1 mol% organocatalyst **2**.

Currently, the use of water as reaction medium has been regarded as a goal in modern organic chemistry due to its cost, safety, and environmentally benign concerns [9]. The pioneer work of organocatalyzed direct aldol reaction in water has been independently reported by Hayashi [10] and Barbas [11]. Then many efforts have been devoted to asymmetric organocatalytic reactions performed in aqueous media [12]. For example, Singh and co-workers reported L-prolineamide organocatalyst 11 for the direct asymmetric aldol reaction of ketone with aldehyde acceptor in excellent enantioselectivity and with low catalyst loading (0.5-1 mol%) in aqueous media (Figure 6) [13]. Gryko employed 2.5-10 mol% L-prolinethioamide to effectively catalyze the aldol reaction of cyclohexanone and aromatic aldehydes in the presence of water [14].

To the best of our knowledge, as for the acyclic acetone as a donor, there were few reports about the direct asymmetric aldol reaction carried out in water compared to cyclic ketone. Consequently, it still remains a challenge to develop high efficient organocatalysts for the direct asymmetric aldol reactions of acetone and aromatic aldehydes in water with the amount of organocatalysts as low as possible [15].

The fine adjustment of catalyst structure may cause large affection for the asymmetric reaction. Considering this, we tried to introduce two phenyl groups to change the primary alcohol of the catalyst 1 to tert-alcohol 2 so as to increase the liposolubility (Figure 6). This aqueous reaction is in fact interfacial of water reaction. After optimizing the reaction conditions, we found employing only 0.2 mol% amount of catalyst 2, the reaction could be performed efficiently in water and obtain the excellent yields' and excellent enantioselectivities' hydroxyl carbonyl compounds for almost all aldehydes substrates (Table 1).

It is well-known that the aldol reaction of hydroxyacetone is a versatile route to construct the 1,2-diol building blocks for the synthesis of various natural and biological active molecules [16].

To further evaluate the prolinethioamide catalysts synthesized by us and as a continuous of our work on the asymmetric reaction, we selected the aldol reaction of hydroxyacetone and p-nitrobenzaldehyde as a model reaction. Interestingly, two chemselective diol products 13 and 14 could be obtained when screening the various organocatalysts. For example, in the presence of dipeptide derivatives, not only 1,2-diol was obtained but also 1,4 diol produced with high enantioselectivities, respectively. This case excites our interests to give an insight study if high chemselective single product could be obtained by control the reaction conditions.

Table 2. Screening the various organocatalyst in the direct asymmetric aldol reactions of hydroxyacetone with *p*-nitrobenzaldehyde [a]

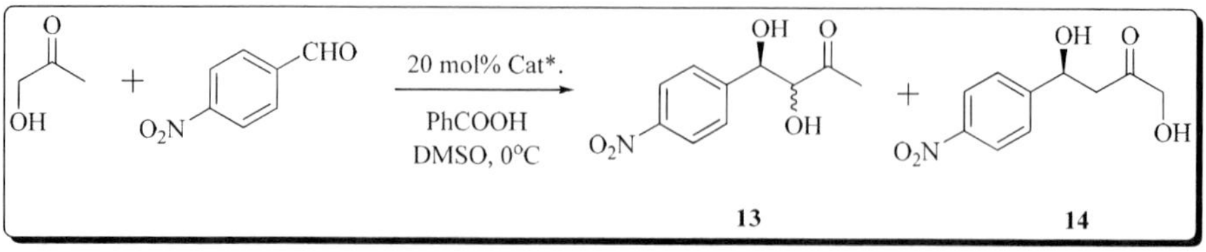

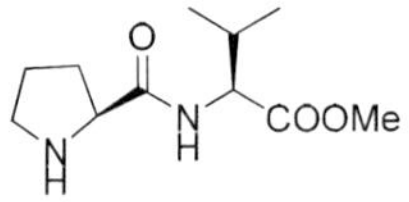

15

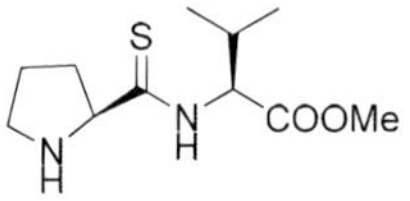

3

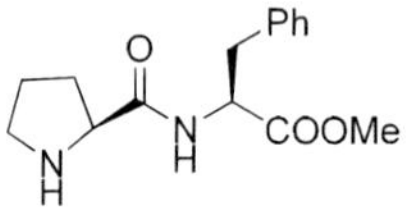

16

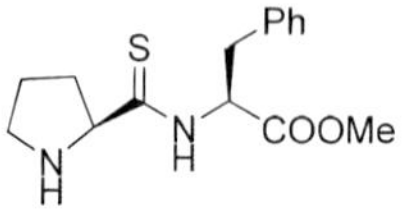

17

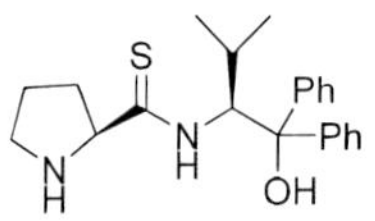

2

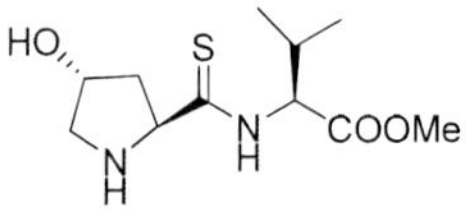

18

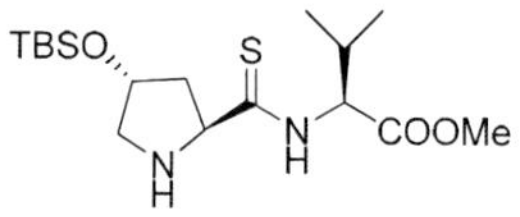

19

Entry	Cat*	13			14	
		Syn: anti	Yield (%)	ee (%)	Yield (%)	ee (%)
1	**15**	7:3	89	50	-	-
2	**3**	**8:1**	**67**	**88**	**21**	**94**
3	**16**	7:3	86			
4	**17**	8:2	80			
5	**2**	-	<10	-	-	-
6	**18**	2.8	75	33	16	-
7	**19**	5:1	62	11	25	82

Through the great amount of reaction conditions examinations (Table 3), to our delighted, we found an optimal protocol in which two products could be respectively obtained with moderate or high yield and high enantioselectivity in the presence of the same organocatalyst with only different additives (Scheme 7).

Table 3. The different additives screening employed in the direct asymmetric aldol reaction of hydroxyacetone with *p*-nitrobenzaldehyde

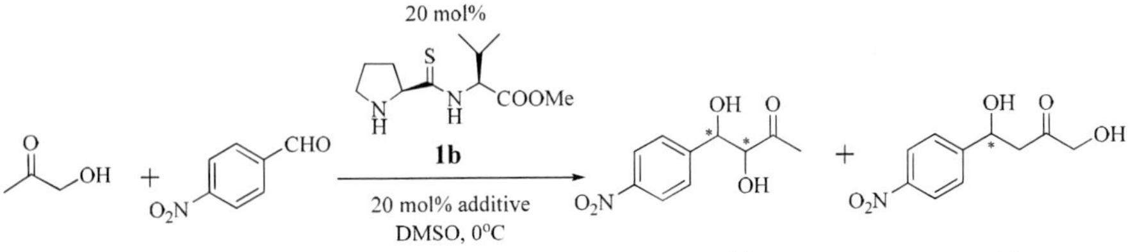

13 **1,2-diol product** **14** **1,4-diol product**

Entry	Additive	Product 13 Yield(%)[a]	anti:syn[b]	ee(%)[c]	Product 14 Yield(%)[a]	ee(%)[c]	Total Yield(%)[c]
1	-	65	8:2	79	22	90	87
2	PhCOOH	67	8:1	88	21	94	88
3	2-OH-C_6H_4COOH	86	8:1	89	-	-	86
4	4-OH-C_6H_4COOH	27	7:1	65	50	90	77
5	Phthalic acid	65	8:1	67	29	90	94
6	PhOH	27	1:1	50	30	91	57
7	2-OH-C_6H_4OH	45	1:1	47	54	90	99
8	R-Binol	62	8:2	50	25	86	87
9	Al_2O_3	6	9:1	63	67	93	73
10	Al_2O_3+5 uL H_2O	12	8:1	30	64	92	76
11	Al_2O_3(basic)	38	8:2	43	50	98	88
12	SiO_2	55	4:1	56	44	90	99
13	ZnO	37	6:1	67	63	85	100
14	MgO	47	7:1	7	25	89	72
15	CaO	20	1:9	10	21	93	41

[a] Isolated yield□[b] the diastereoselectivity value was determined by the H NMR, [c] The ee was determined by HPLC using a chiral stationary phase (Daicel Chiralpak AD-H or AS-H).

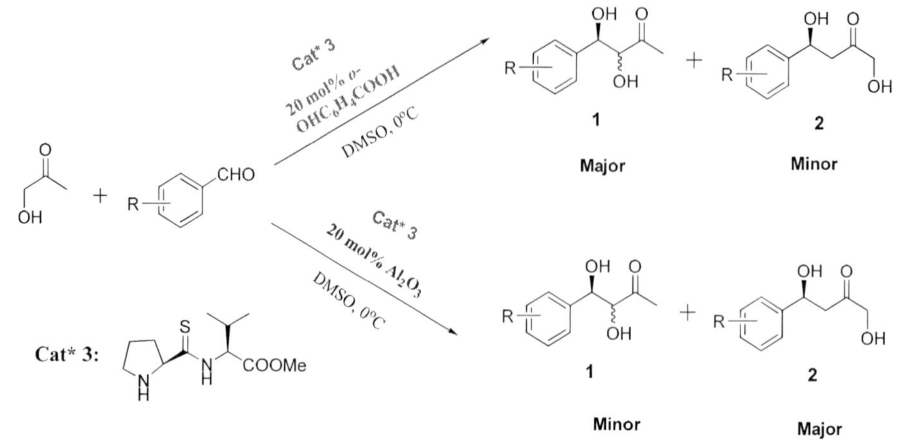

Scheme 7. The regioselective asymmetric aldol reaction of hydroxyacetone and *p*-nitrobenzaldehyde.

2.3. The Application of Organocatalysts Derived from the L-Proline in the Asymmetric Allylation Reaction of Aldehydes

The asymmetric allylation of carbonyl compounds has become one of the most useful methods for the formation of carbon-carbon bond in modern organic synthesis. This reaction could furnish chiral homoallylic alcohols products which are the versatile intermediates for the synthesis of many natural products and pharmaceuticals [17]. Therefore, there has been an intense research activity in this area in recent years, and then leading to the development of chiral catalysts [18]. Among these approaches, most reports mainly focus on the chiral metal complexes which are generally sensitive to the air and moisture (combining metal Lewis acid with the chiral ligand). Moreover, in previously reported catalytic asymmetric allylations of aldehydes, allylstannane such as allyl-tributyltin, tetra-allyltin or trimethylallylsilane is usually used. In these cases, only the allyl group could reappear in the product and thus there is no atom economy. Recently, there are some reports about the asymmetric allylation of allyltrichlorosilane and aldehydes catalyzed by the Lewis base metal complexes [19].

On the other hand, the Barbier-type coupling reaction between allyl halide and carbonyl compounds promoted by low valent metal tin, indium or its halides has been developed to be an efficient way to prepare homoallylic alcohols over the past few decades, and has received more and more attention due to its suitable activity, low cost and low toxicity of the final inorganic tin derivatives. Such reactions are believed to involve in the situ formation of solvated monoallyltin trihalides or diallyltin dihalides as active allyltin species. With respect to this, our group began to study the asymmetric allylation of aldehydes promoted by an L-proline derivative in the presence of Lewis base, using the allyltin tribromide, which acts not only as an allyl group donor but also as an intrinsic Lewis acid combining with the chiral ligand (Scheme 8). This reaction will hopefully establish the groundwork for the Barbier-type asymmetric allylation of aldehydes with organotin reagents.

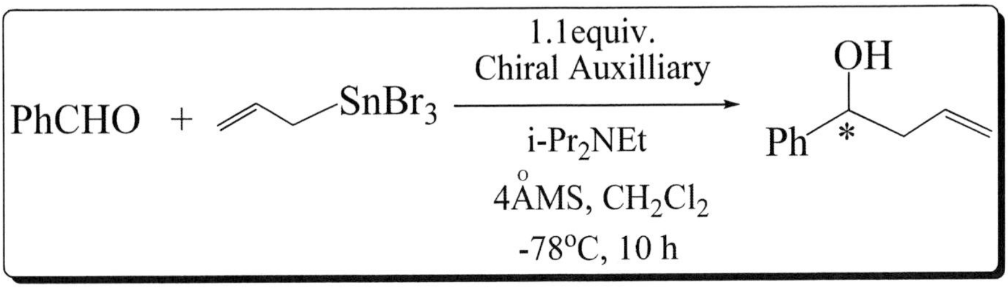

Scheme 8. The asymmetric allylation of aldehyde.

Selecting a suitable chiral catalyst is the important key point for an asymmetric reaction. Thus, a series of various proline derivatives were examined firstly in our initial study (Figure 7). It could be observed that the organocatalyst D was the best chiral source. On the basis of this, we expand our optimal protocol to the various aldehydes (Figure 8).

Asymmetric organocatalysis based on either Lewis acid or base has been recognized as an efficient method for obtaining chiral compounds with high enantioselectivity. The application of enantiomerically pure 'small' organic molecules represents a promising alternative catalytic concept in addition to the frequently used metal complexes catalysts [20]. Yanagisawa reported the asymmetric allylation of aldehydes with tetraallyltin catalyzed by L-aspartic acid in 2004, but the best enantiomeric excess value was only 40% [21]. In addition, Tsogoeva et. al published allylation of imine catalyzed by chiral formamide derivatives with the participation of 2 equiv. L-proline in 2006 [22]. Obviously, there was a double molecule chiral catalysis in this reaction. On the basis of these concepts, and as continuation of our ongoing program on asymmetric allylation of carbonyl compounds catalyzed by small organic molecules, we herein found an asymmetric allylation of aldehydes using triallyltin monobromide catalyzed by double small organic molecules such as natural L-proline and L-prolinol, which are widely used owing to availability, stability and low cost. Similarly, various reaction parameters were tested including chiral auxiliaries or theirs amounts and allyltin reagents. Finally, the various aldehydes were investigated in the optimized reaction conditions (Table 4).

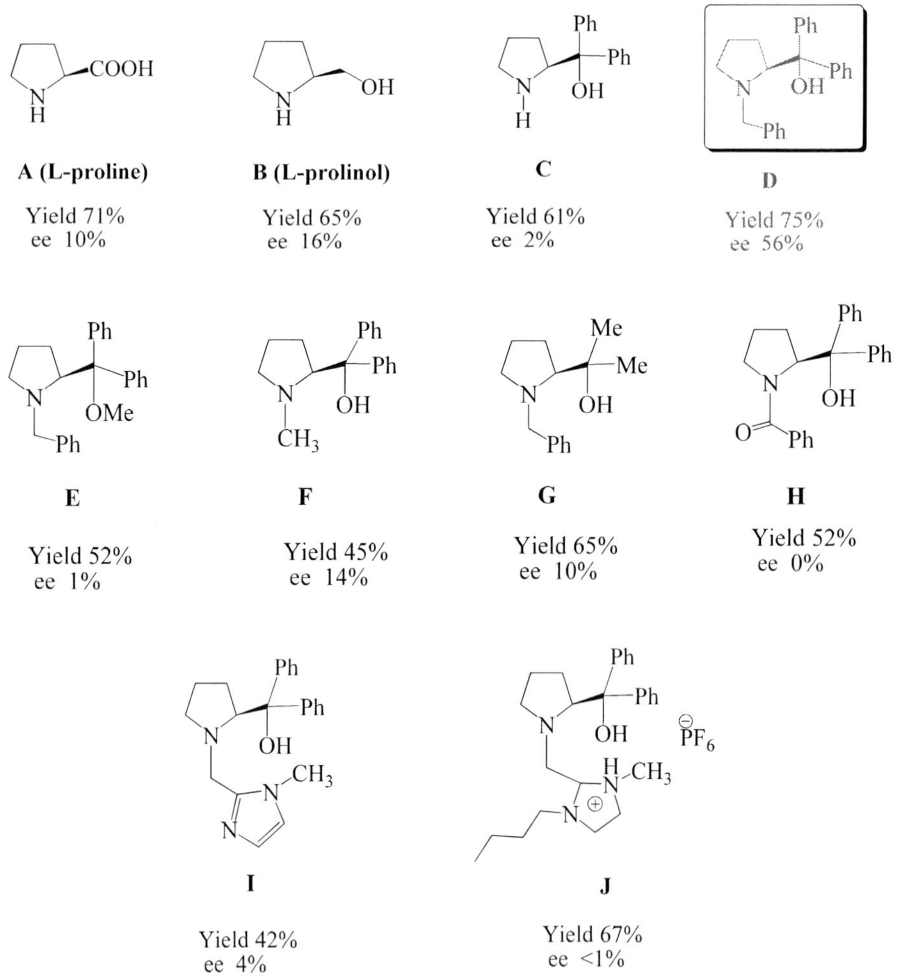

Figure 7. various proline derivatives employed in the asymmetric allylation of benzaldehyde and tribromoallyltin.

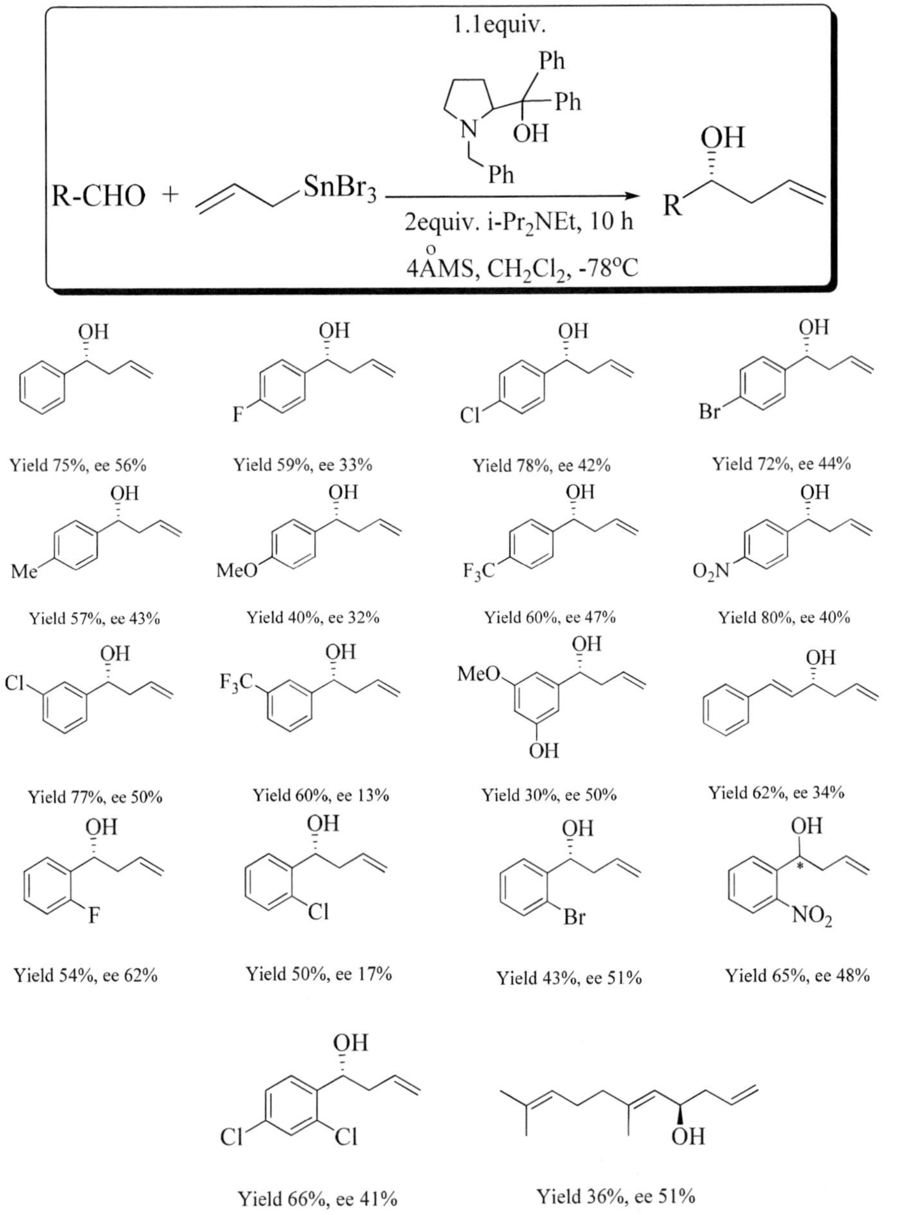

Figure 8. The corresponding chiral homoallyl alcohols.

Table 4. The asymmetric allylation of triallyltin monobromide with various aldehydes

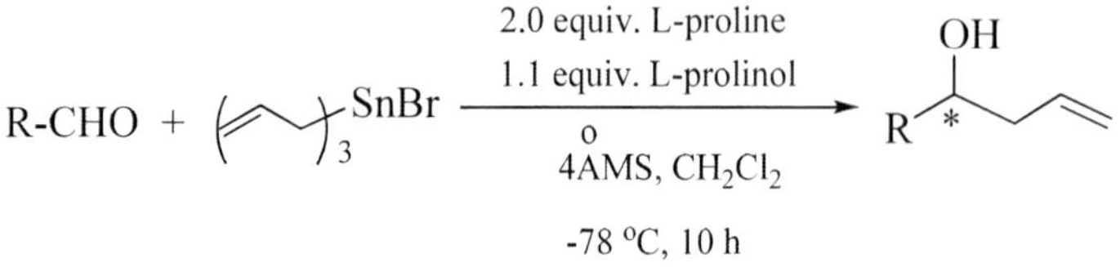

Entry	R	Yield/%[a]	ee/%[b]	Config.[c]
1	Ph	86	56	R
2	*p*-ClC_6H_4	89	62	R
3	*p*-BrC_6H_4	87	64	R
4	*p*-$CF_3C_6H_4$	83	59	R
5	*p*-$NO_2C_6H_4$	-	-	-
6	*p*-MeC_6H_4	72	57	R
7	*p*-$MeOC_6H_4$	78	59	R
8	*o*-FC_6H_4	82	42	R
9	*o*-BrC_6H_4	88	40	R
10	*o*-$NO_2C_6H_4$	86	46	R
11	*o*-$CF_3C_6H_4$	85	35	R
12	*m*-BrC_6H_4	90	47	R
13	*m*-$NO_2C_6H_4$	74	50	R
14	*m*-CF_3 C_6H_4	89	46	R
15	*2,4-dichloro*C_6H_3	84	32	R
16	Ph-CH=CH-	61	54	R
17	CH_3-CH=CH-	14	4	R
18	heptanal	<10	-	-

[a] Isolated yield, [b] Chiral GC (γ-cyclodextrin column), [c] The absolute configuration of the product was determined by comparison of the optical rotation with literatures.

2.4. The Application of Organocatalysts Derived from the L-Proline in the Allylation Reaction or Ring-opening of Epoxides

Epoxides are the most useful and versatile substrates in organic synthesis due to their high reactivity [23-28]. A number of methods have been reported for the cleavage of epoxides with various nucleophiles, such as carbon-based nucleophiles [29-30], halides [31], alcohols [32-33] and so on. The corresponding β-substituted alcohols products are widely applied in the synthesis of natural products and pharmaceuticals [34]. However, only a few methods are known for the allylation of epoxides with allylmetal reagents. For example, allyl magnesium, allyl zinc and allylsilane are widely employed in the last century [35-37]. Recently, the applications of allylstannane in the allylation of epoxides are reported. [38-40]. And these methods suffer from a lack of efficiency and simplicity. Therefore, the development of simple and novel reagents, which are more efficient and provide convenient procedures with improved yields and high regioselectivity still remains a challenge for synthetic organic chemists. In continuation of our ongoing program on the allylation of carbonyl compound mediated by organotin reagent [41], we studied the further application of organotin reagents [42-43]. Herein, we described the ring opening reaction of epoxides with allyltin tribromides as a new alternative method for allylation in the presence of L-proline 4. Simultaneously, we observed a byproduct with high yield—halohydrin when the reaction conditions were screened. The allyltin tribromide can react with epoxide and give the halohydrins in high yields with complete regioselectivity catalyzed by the L-proline derivative 6. In addition, it can also act as a Lewis acid to catalyze the ring opening reactions of epoxides with alcohols (Scheme 8).

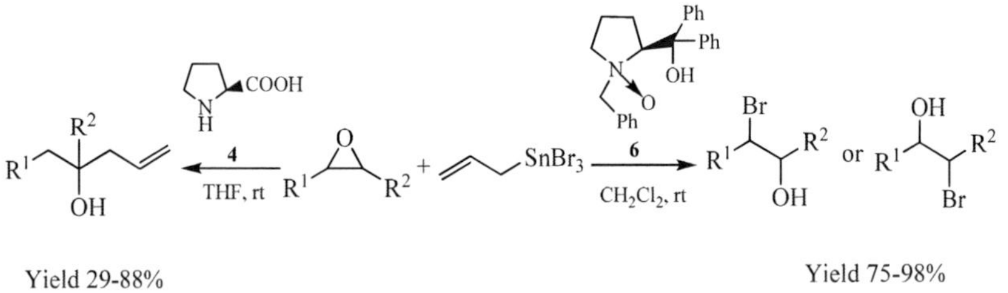

Scheme 8. The allylation reaction or ring-opening of epoxides catalyzed by the L-proline or its derivative

2.5. The Application of Organocatalysts Derived from the L-Proline in the Asymmetric Michael Addition Reaction of cycloketones and chalcones

The Michael addition reaction is widely considered as one of the most important carbon-carbon bond-forming reactions in organic synthesis [44]. Among them, the Michael addition of cyclic ketones to active acceptors, such as cyclohexanone and nitroolefin, has attracted intense attention over the past decade [45]. And so far there have been lots of successful reports [45-46]. In comparison, asymmetric Michael addition reactions of cyclic ketones and low reactive α,β-unsaturated ketones, namely chalcones, are few reported and still remains a major challenge. For example, Wang Wei research group used a chiral pyrrolidinylmethylsulfonamide as an organocatalyst for the Michael addition of cyclohexanone to chalcones and got the desired products with the moderate yields (65%-85%), good enantioselectivities (≥90%) and diastereo- meric ratios (>50:1) [47] But this reaction is generally completed in a long time (more than 4 days) in the presence of this organocatalyst. And then Wang Yongmei and co-workers reported the Michael addition of cyclohexanone to chalcones catalyzed by the pyrrolidine-pyridine base, chiral pyrrolidine-phosphite organocatalyst or amino acid ionic liquid [EMIm][Pro], respectively, and obtained the corresponding products with the good yields and enantioselectivities as well as excellent diastereomeric ratios [48]. Nevertheless, in the case of cyclopentanone, this Michael addition reaction with chalcone gave the adducts with only moderate level of ee value under the same protocol. Recently, Li *et al.*, employed the pyrrolidine-based imides to catalyze the Michael addition of cyclic ketones to chalcones, while the 30 mol% catalyst was used and the longer time 7 days was necessary for the reaction [49]. Therefore, the development of more highly efficient organocatalysts for the Michael addition of low reactive chalcones to the cyclic ketones is an urgent and of great significant. Moreover, as far as the Michael addition reaction of cyclopentanone with chalcone is concerned, the reports are very fewer than that of cyclohexanone [47-51]. It may be due to the low reactivity and high steric hinderance of chalcone as well as the cyclopentanone's high tension. In view of this, achieving the broad substrates and higher selectivity intrigued our interests. Our research group developed the organophosphine catalyst [52] derived from L-proline for catalyzing the asymmetric Michael addition of cyclic ketones to chalcones (Scheme 9). As a result, we found two optimal system suitable for the Michael reaction of cyclohexanone or cyclopentanone with chalcones, respectively (Figure 9).

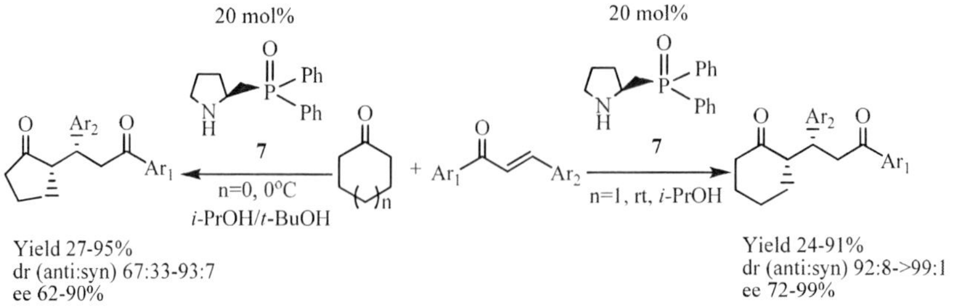

Scheme 9. The asymmetric Michael addition reaction of cycloketones and chalcones.

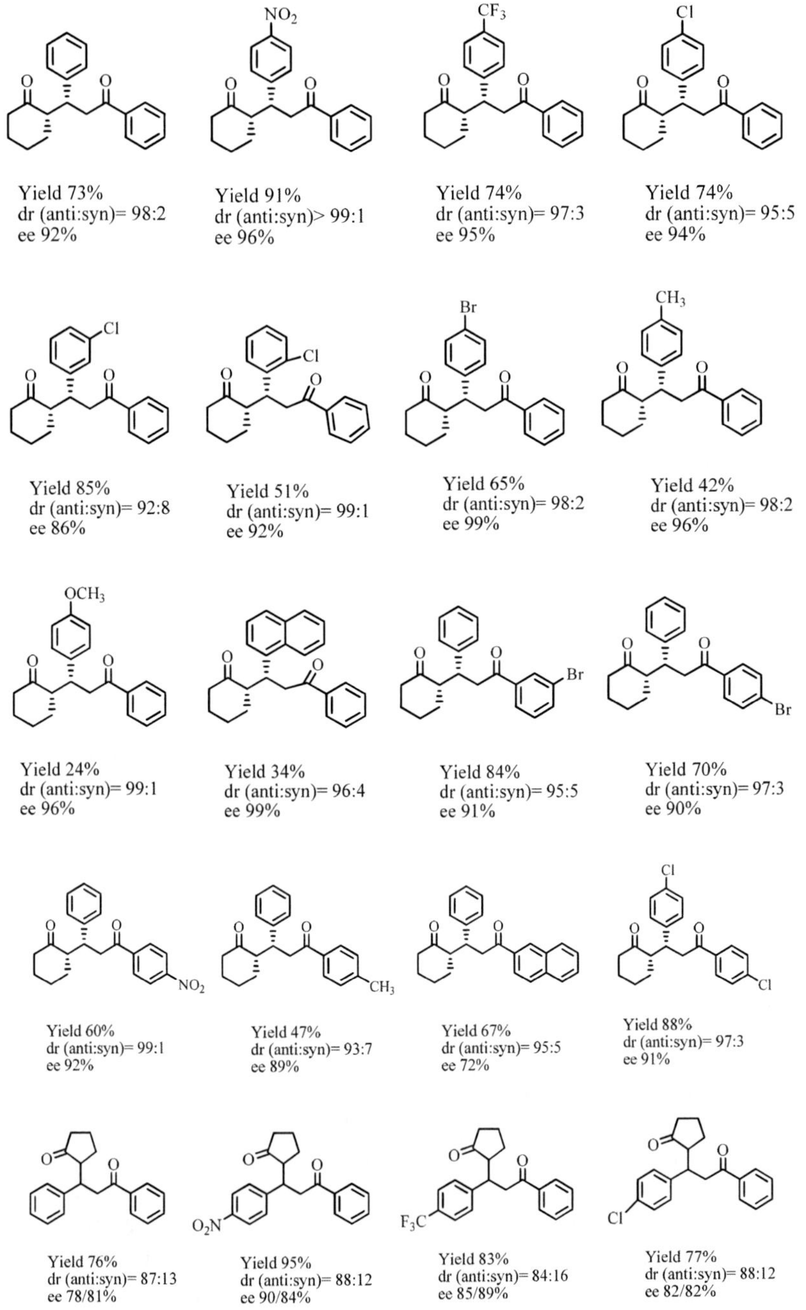

Figure 9 (Continued).

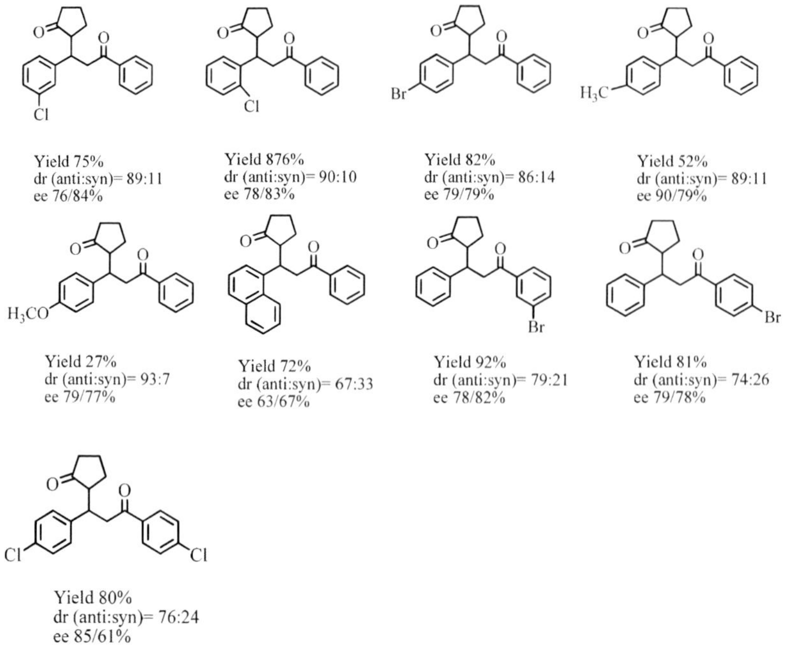

Figure 9. The corresponding Michael products.

In conclusion, the field of organocatalysis has received considerable attention in the past decades. The efficiency and the scope of organocatalytic reactions have been broadly established. In this area, enamine catalysis or iminium catalysis is one of the most studied activate intermediate which allows aldol reactions, Mannich reactions, Michael additions, cycloadditions and many other transformations with excellent selectivities.

References

[1] Z. G. Hajos, D. R. Parrish, *J. Org. Chem.* 1974, 39, 1615.

[2] B. List, *J. Am. Chem. Soc.* 2000, 122, 9336.

[3] a) A. Dondon, A. Massi, *Angew. Chem. Int. Ed.* 2008, *47*, 4638; b) B. List, J. W. Yang, *Science*, 2006, *313*, 1584; c) D. W. C. MacMillan, *Nature*, 2008, *455*, 304; d) P. I. Dalko, Enantioselective Organocatalysis: Reactions and Experimental Procedures, Wiley-VCH, Weinheim, 2007; e) M. J. Gaunt, C. C. C. Johansson, A. McNally, N. C. Vo, *Drug Discovery Today*, 2007, *12*, 8; e) A. Berkessel, H. Groger, Asymmetric Organocatalysis-From

Biomimetic Concepts to Powerful Methods for Asymmetric Synthesis, Wiley-VCH, Weinheim, 2005; f) J. Seayad, B. List, *Org. Biomol. Chem.* 2005, *3*, 719; g) P. I. Dalko, L. Moisan, *Angew. Chem. Int. Ed.* 2004, 43, 5138.

[4] a) P. Melchiorre, M. Marigo, A. Carlone and G. Bartoli, *Angew. Chem. Int. Ed.* 2008, *47*, 6138; b) F.-Z. Peng, Z.-H. Shao, *J. Mol. Catal. A: Chem.* 2008, *285*, 1; c) C. F. Barbas III, *Angew. Chem. Int. Ed.* 2008, 47, 42; d) B. List, *Chem. Commun.* 2006, 819; e) M. Marigo, K. A. Jorgensen, *Chem. Commun.* 2006, 2001; f) A. J. A. Cobb, D. M. Shaw, D. A. Longbottom, J. B. Gold, S. V. Ley, *Org. Biomol. Chem.* 2005, 3, 84; g) W. Notz, F. Tanaka, C. F. Barbas III, *Acc. Chem. Res.* 2004, *37*, 580; h) E. R. Jarvo, S. J. Miller, *Tetrahedron*, 2002, *58*, 2481; i) B. List, *Synlett*, 2001, 1675; j) S. Mukherjee, J. W. Yang, S. Hoffmann, B. List, *Chem. Rev.* 2007, 107, 5471; k) B. List, *Acc. Chem. Res.* 2004, 37, 548; l) A. ErkkilV, I. Majander and P. M. Pihko, *Chem. Rev.* 2007, 107, 5416; m) G. Lelais, D. W. C. MacMillan, *Aldrichimica Acta*, 2006, 39, 79; n) X.-H. Yu, W. Wang, *Chem.-Asian J.* 2008, *3*, 516; o) S. J. Connon, *Chem. Commun.* 2008, 2499; p) A. G. Doyle, E. N. Jacobsen, *Chem. Rev.* 2007, 107, 5713; q) T. Akiyama, *Chem. Rev.* , 2007, *107*, 5744; r) Y. Takemoto, H. Miyabe, *Chimia* 2007, 61, 269; s) M. S. Taylor, E. N. Jacobsen, *Angew. Chem. Int. Ed.* 2006, 45, 1520; t) S. J. Connon, *Chem.–Eur. J.* 2006, *12*, 5418; u) S. J. Connon, *Angew. Chem. Int. Ed.* 2006, *45*, 3909; v) Y. Takemoto, *Org. Biomol. Chem.* 2005, *3*, 4299; w) C. Bolm, T. Rantanen, I. Schiffers, L. Zani, *Angew. Chem. Int. Ed.* 2005, *44*, 1758; x) P. M. Pihko, *Angew. Chem. Int. Ed.* 2004, *43*, 2062; y) P. R. Schreiner, *Chem. Soc. Rev.* 2003, 32, 289; z) T. Ooi, K. Maruoka, *Angew. Chem., Int. Ed.* 2007, *46*, 4222; aa) M. O'Donnell, *Acc. Chem. Res.* 2004, *37*, 506; ab) B. Lygo, B. I. Andrews, *Acc. Chem. Res.* 2004, 37, 518; ac) K. Maruoka and T. Ooi, *Chem. Rev.* 2003, *103*, 3013; ad) T. Marcelli, T. H. van Maarseveen and H. Hiemstra, *Angew. Chem. Int. Ed.* 2006, 45, 7496; ae) S.-K. Tian, Y. Chen, J. Hang, L. Tang, P. McDaid, L. Deng, *Acc. Chem. Res.* 2004, 37, 621; af) S. France, D. J. Guerin, S. J. Miller and T. Letcka, *Chem. Rev.* 2003, 103, 2985.

[5] Z. Tang, L.-Z. Gong, *J. Am. Chem. Soc.* 2003, 125, 5262.

[6] a) Z. Tang, L.-Z.Gong, *J. Am. Chem. Soc.* 2005, 127, 9285; b) L. He, Z. Tang, L.-Z. Gong, *Tetrahedron* 2006, 62, 346; c) G. Luppi, *Tetrahedron* 2006, *62*, 12017; d) M. Raj, S. K. Ginotra, V. K. Singh, *Org. Lett* 2006, 8, 4097; e) V. Maya, M. Raj, V. K. Singh, *Org. Lett.* 2007, 9, 2593; f) R. S. Rambo, P. H. Schneider, *Tetrahedron: Asymmetry* 2010, 21, 2254; g) G. R. Dorota, *Adv. Synth. Catal.* 2005, 347, 1948; h) D. Gryko, *J. Org. Chem.*

2007, *72*, 964; i) D. Alma, C. Najera, *Adv. Synth. Catal.* 2008, 350, 2467; j) B. K. Albrecht, L. Johann, *Adv. Synth. Catal.* 2004, 346, 1141; k) A. J. A. Cobb, D. M. Shaw, D. A. Longbottom, J. B. Gold, S. V. Ley, *Org. Biomol. Chem.* 2005, *3*, 84; l) F. Silva, M. Sawicki, V. Gouverneur, *Org. Lett.* 2006, 8, 5417; m) Y. Wu, Y. Zhang, M. Yu, G. Zhao, S. Wang, *Org. Lett.* 2006, 8, 4417; n) J.-R. Chen, J. Wan, W.-J. Xiao, *Org. Lett.* 2005, 7, 4543; o) S. Samanta, J. Liu, R. Dodda, C.-G. Zhao, *Org. Lett.* 2005, 7, 5321; p) F. Wang, Y. Xiong, X. Feng, *Adv Synth Catal.* 2007, 349, 2665; q) Y.-N. Jia, C.-S. Da, *Tetrahedron Lett.* 2009, *50*, 3059; r) G. Guillena,; M. D. C. Hita, C. Najera, S. F. Viozquez, *J. Org. Chem.* 2008, 73, 5933; s) S. Guizzetti, M. Benaglia, *Tetrahedron: Asymmetry* 2006, 17, 2754; t) S. Guizzetti, M. Benaglia, *Org. Lett.* 2007, *9*, 1247; u) M. K. Zhu, L. F. Cun, A. Q. Mi, Y. Z. Jiang, L. Z. Gong, *Tetrahedron: Asymmetry* 2006, 17, 491; v) M. Jiang, S. F. Zhu, L. Z. Gong, Q. L. Zhou, *Tetrahedron: Asymmetry* 2006, 17, 384; w) J.-R. Chen, X.-L. An, X.-Y. Zhu, X.-F. Wang, W.-J.Xiao, *J. Org. Chem.* 2008, 73, 6006.

[7] a) B. Wang, L. Y. Liu, W. X. Chang, J. Li, *Adv. Synth. Catal.* 2009, *351*, 2441; b) B. Wang, L. Y. Liu, W. X. Chang, J. Li, *Eur. J. Org. Chem.* 2010, 31, 5951.

[8] a) G. Casiraghi, F. Zanardi, G. Appendino, G. Rassu, *Chem. Rev.* 2000, 100, 1929; b) T. D. Machajewski, C. H. Wong, *Angew. Chem. Int. Ed.* 2000, 39, 1352.

[9] a) M. Benaglia, M. Cinquini, F. Cozzi, G. Celentano, *Org. Biomol. Chem.* 2004, *2,* 3401; b) R. Mestres, *Green Chem.* 2004, *6*, *583*.

[10] a) Y. Hayashi, T. Sumiya, J. Takahashi, H. Gotoh, T. Urushima, M. Shoji, *Angew. Chem. Int. Ed.* 2006, 45, 958; b) S. Aratake, T. Itoh, T. Okano, T. Usui, M. Shoji, Y. Hayashi, *Chem. Commun.* 2007, 2524; c) S. Aratake, T. Itoh, T. Okano, N. Nagae, T. Sumiya, M. Shoji, Y. Hayashi, *Chem.-Eur. J.* 2007, 13, 10246.

[11] a) A. Cordova, W. Notz, C. F. Barbas, *Chem. Commun.* 2002, 3024; b) N. Mase, Y. Nakai, N. Ohara, H. Yoda, K. Takabe, F. Tanaka, C. F. Barbas, *J. Am. Chem. Soc.* 2006, 128, 734; c) S. S. V. Ramasastry, H. Zhang, F. Tanaka, C. F. III. Barbas, *J. Am. Chem. Soc.* 2007, 129, 288.

[12] a) Y. Watanabe, K. Sawada, M. Hayashi, *Green Chem.* 2010, 12, 384; b) S. S. V. Ramasastry, K. Albertshofer, N. Utsumi, C. F. Barbas, *Org. Lett.* 2008, 10, 1621; c) S. Guizzetti, M. Benaglia, L. Raimondi, G. Celentano, *Org. Lett.* 2007, *9*, 1247; d) M. Lei, L. X. Shi, G. Li, S. Chen, W. H. Fang, Z. M. Ge, T. M. Cheng,R. T. Li, *Tetrahedron* 2007, 63, 7892; e) J. F. Zhao, L. He, J. Jiang, Z. Tang, L. F. Cun, L. Z. Gong, *Tetrahedron Lett.* 2008, 49,

3372; f) S. S. Chimni, S. Singh, D. Mahajan, *Tetrahedron: Asymmetry* 2008, 19, 2276; g) Z. Jiang, H. Yang, X. Han, J. Luo, M. W. Wong, Y. Lu, *Org. Biomol. Chem.* 2010, *8*, 1368; h) M. Gruttadauria, *Eur. J. Org. Chem.* 2009, 5437.

[13] a) M. Raj, G. Parashari and V. Singh, *Adv. Synth. Catal.* 2009, *351*, 1284; b) V. Maya, M. Raj, V. K. Singh, *Org. Lett.* 2007, 9, 2593; c) M. Raj, Vishnumaya, S. K. Ginotra ,V. K. Singh, *Org. Lett.* 2006, 8, 4097.

[14] a) D. Gryko, M. Zimnicka, R. Lipinski, *J. Org. Chem.* 2007, 72, 964; b) D. Gryko, W. J. Saletra, *Org. Biomol. Chem.* 2007, 5, 2148.

[15] a) Y. N. Jia, F. C. Wu, X. Ma, G. J. Zhu, C. S. Da, *Tetrahedron Lett.* 2009, 50, 3059; b) M. Jiang, S. F. Zhu, Y. Yang, L. Z. Gong, X. G. Zhou, Q. L. Zhou, *Tetrahedron: Asymmetry* 2006, 17, 384.

[16] For reviews, see: a) K. C. Nicolaou, S. A. Snyder, Classics in Total Synthesis II ; Wiley-VCH: Weinheim, Germany, 2003; b) N. Yoshikawa, N. Kumagai, S. Matsunaga, G. Moll, T. Ohshima, T. Suzuki, M. Shibasaki, *J. Am. Chem. Soc.* 2001, 123, 2466; c) N. Kumagai, S. Matsunaga, T. Kinoshita, S. Harada, S. Okada, S. Sakamoto, K. Yamaguchi, M. Shibasaki, *J. Am. Chem. Soc.* 2003, 125, 2169; d) B. M. Trost, H. Ito, E. R. Silcoff, *J. Am. Chem. Soc.* 2001, 123, 3367; e) D. Shabat, B. List, R. A. Lerner, C. F. Barbas III, *Tetrahedron Lett.* 1999, 40, 1437; f) B. List, D. Shabat, C. F. Barbas III, R. A. Lerner, *Chem. Eur. J.* 1999, *4*, 881; g) D. Xu, G. A. Crispino, K. B. Sharpless, *J. Am. Chem. Soc.* 1992, 114, 7570; h) H. C. Kolb, P. G. Andersson, K. B. Sharpless, *J. Am. Chem. Soc.* 1994, 116, 1278; i) W. Notz, B. List, *J. Am. Chem. Soc.* 2000, 122, 7386.

[17] a) S. E. Denmark, J.-P. Fu, *Chem. Rev.* 2003, 103, 2763; b) K. C. Nicolaou, D. W. Kim, R. Baati, *Angew. Chem. Int. Ed.* 2002, 41, 3701; c) M. Shi, G.-X. Lei, Y. Masaki, *Tetrahedron: Asymmetry.* 1999, *10*, 2071; d) Y. Wang, B.-M. Ji, K.-L. Ding, *Chin. J. Chem.* 2002, 20, 1300; e) Z.-G. Zha, Z. Xie, C.-L. Zhou, Z.-Y. Wang, Y.-S. Wang, *Chin. J. Chem.* 2002, 20, 1477.

[18] For some examples see: a) G. E. Keck, K. H. Tarbet, L. S. Geraci, *J. Am. Chem. Soc.* 1993, 115, 8467; b) A. L. Cosata, M. G. Piazza, E. Tagliavini, C. Trombini, A. U. Ronchi, *J. Am. Chem. Soc.*, 1993, 115, 7001; c) Yanagisawa, A.; Nakashima, H.; Ishiba, A.; H. Yamamoto, *J. Am. Chem. Soc.* 1996, 118, 4723; d) A. Yana-gisawa, A. Ishiba, H. Nakashima, H. Yamamoto, *Synlett*, 1996, 88; e) A. Yanagisawa, H. Nakashima, Y. Nakatsuka, A. Ishiba, H. Yamamoto, *Bull. Chem. Soc. Jpn.* 2001, 74, 1129; f) H. Hanawa, T. Hashimoto, K. Maruoka, *J. Am. Chem. Soc.* 2003, *125*, 1708; g) P. G. Cozzi, P. Orioli, E. Tagliavini, A. Umani-Ronchi,

Tetrahedron Lett. 1997, 38, 145; h) T.-P. Loh, In Science of Synthesis; H. Yamamoto, Ed.; Georg Thieme Verlag Stutt-gart: New York, 2004, 413.

[19] a) A. Massa, A. V. Malkov, P. Kocovsky, et al. *Tetrahedron Lett.* 2003, 44: 7179; b) R. M. Angell, A. G. M. Barrett, B. D. Vickery, et al. *Chem. Commun.* 1997, 919; c) I. Chataigner, U. Piarulli, C. Gennari, *Tetrahedron Lett.* 1999, 40, 3633; d) M, Nakajima, S, Kotani, S, Hashimoto, et al. *Tetrahedron Lett.* 2005, *46*, 157; e) S. Kobayashi, K. Nishio, *Tetrahedron Lett.* 1993, 34, 3453.

[20] a) H. Gröger, J. Wilken, *Angew. Chem. Int. Ed.* 2001, *40*, 529; b) B. List, *Synlett* 2001, 1675; c) E. Jarvo, S. Miller, *Tetrahedron* 2002, 58, 2481; d) B. List, *Tetrahedron* 2002, *58*, 5573.

[21] A. Yanagisawa, Y. Nakamura, T. Arai, *Tetrahedron: Asymmetry* 2004, 15, 1909.

[22] S. Jagtap, S. Tsogoeva, *Chem. Commun.* 2006, 4747.

[23] C. Bonini, G. Righi, *Synthesis,* 1994, 225.

[24] N. Iranpoor, I. M. Baltork Mild, *Synth. Commun.* 1990, 20, 2789.

[25] M. Shimizu, A. Yoshida, T. Fujisawa, *Synlett,* 1992, 3, 204.

[26] S. Munavalli, D. K. Rohrbaugh, H. D. Durst, et al. *Phosphorus, Sulfur, and Silicon and the Related Elements,* 2002, 177, 215.

[27] D. Rix, F. Caijo, M. Mauduit, et al. *J. Org. Chem.* 2008, 73, 4225.

[28] Y. Usami, K. Mizuki, H. Ichikawa, M. Arimoto, *Tetrahedron: Asymmetry,* 2008, 19, 1461.

[29] M. Lautens, M. L. Maddess, E. L. O. Sauer, S. G. Ouellet, *Org. Lett.* 2002, 4, 83.

[30] P. Mauro, *Eur. J. Org. Chem.* 2006, 22, 4979.

[31] C. D. Roy, *Austr. J. Chem.* 2006, 59, 834.

[32] M. W. C. Robinson, R. Buckle, I. Mabbett, G. M. Grant, A. E. Graham, *Tetrahedron Lett.* 2007, 48, 4723.

[33] D. Jiang, A. Urakawa, M. Yulikov, A. Baiker, et al. *Chem. Eur. J.* 2009, 15, 12255.

[34] I. Cabanal-Duvillard, J. F. Berrien, H. P. Husson, et al. *Tetrahedron Lett.* 1998, 39, 5181.

[35] D. F. Taber, J. H. Green, J. M. Geremia. *J. Orga. Chem.* 1997, 62, 9342.

[36] D. Abenhaim, E. Henry-Basch, P. Freon, *Comptes Rendus des Seances de l'Academie des Sciences, Serie C Sciences Chimiques,* 1968, 267, 655.

[37] T. Imai, S. Nishida, *J. Org. Chem.* 1990, 55, 4849.

[38] P. R. Likhar, M. P. Kumar, A. K. Bandyopadhyay, *Tetrahedron Lett.* 2002, 43, 3333.

[39] J. S. Yadav, B. V. S. Reddy, G. Satheesh, *Tetrahedron Lett.* 2003, 44, 6501.

[40] U. K. Roy, S. Roy, *Tetrahedron,* 2006, 62, 678.
[41] L. Y. Liu, J. Sun, J. Li, et al. *Tetrahedron: Asymmetry,* 2007, 18, 710.
[42] R. Qiu, X. Xu, S. Yin, et al. *Chem. Commun.* 2009, 13, 1679.
[43] T. Zhang, M. Shi, M. Zhao, *Tetrahedron,* 2008, 64, 2412.
[44] P. Perlmutter, *Conjugate Addition Reactions in Organic Synthesis, Pergamon, Oxford*, 1992.
[45] J. M. Betancort, K. Sakthivel, R. Thayumanavan, C. F. Barbas ш, *Tetrahedron lett.*, 2001, 42, 4441. b) O. M. Berner, L. Tedeschi, D. Enders, *Eur. J. Org. Chem.* 2002, 1877; c) O. Andrey, A. Alexakis, A. Tomassini, G. Bernardinelli, *Adv. Synth. Catal.* 2004, 346, 1147; d) S. B. Tsogoeva, *Eur. J. Org. Chem,* 2007, 1701; e) C. L. Cao, X. L. Sun, Zhou, J. L.; Tang, Y. *J. Org. Chem.* 2007, 72, 4073; f) Q. Zhu, L. L. Cheng, Y. V. Lu, *Chem. Commun.* 2008, 6315; g) J. Liu, Z. G. Yang, X. H. Liu, et al. *Org. Biomol. Chem.* 2009, 7, 4120; (h) A. D. Lu, R. H. Wu, Z. H. Zhou, et al. *Eur. J. Org. Chem.* 2010, 2057.
[46] a) A. Alexakis, O. Andrey, *Org. Lett.* 2002, 4, 3611; b) Y. Xu, A. Cordova, *Chem. Commun.* 2006, 460; c) S. B. Tsogoeva, S. Wei, *Chem. Commun.* 2006, 1451; d) M. K. Zhu, L. F. Cun, L. Z. Gong et al. *Tetrahedron: Asymmetry* 2006, 17, 491; e) S. V. Pansare, K. Pandya, *J. Am. Chem. Soc.* 2006, 128, 9624; f) B. Tan, X. F. Zeng, Y. P. Lu, G. F. Zhong, et al. *Org. Lett.* 2009, 11, 1927; g) S. Syu, T. T. Kao, W. Lin, *Tetrahedron* 2010, 891; i) S. Chandrasekhar, T. P. Kumar, K. Haribabu, C. R. Reddy, *Tetrahedron: Asymmetry* 2011, 22, 697.
[47] J. Wang, H. Li, L. Zu, W. Wang, *Adv. Synth. Catal.* 2006, 348, 425.
[48] a) D. Z. Xu, S. Shi, Y. J. Liu, Y. M. Wang, *Tetrahedron* 2009, 65, 9344; b) D. Z. Xu, Y. J. Liu, H. Li, Y. M. Wang, *Tetrahedron* 2010, 66, 8890; c) Y. B. Qian, S. Y. Xiao, L. Liu, Y. M. Wang, *Tetrahedron: Asymmetry* 2008, 19, 1515.
[49] H. Y. Xie, S. R. Ban, J. N. Liu, Q. S. Li, *Tetrahedron Lett.* 2012, 53, 3865.
[50] J. F. Wang, X. Wang, Z. M. Ge, T. M. Cheng, R. T. Li, *Chem. Commun.* 2010, 46, 1751.
[51] a) Y. C. Chen, *Synlett* 2008, 1919; b) Y. F. Liu, Y. Wu, Z. H. Zhou, C. C. Tang, et al. *Tetrahedron: Asymmetry* 2011, 22, 476.
[52] a) M. Shi, L. Chen and C. Li, *J. Am. Chem. Soc.* 2005, 127, 3790; b) Y. Q. Fang, E. N. Jacobsen, *J. Am. Chem. Soc.* 2008, 130, 5660; c) Y. Q. Jiang, M. Shi, *J. Am. Chem. Soc.* 2008, 130, 7202.

In: Proline
Editor: Bouzid Nedjimi

ISBN: 978-1-62257-739-2

Chapter IV

Biophysical Studies of Polyproline Peptides

M. Tanty and M-A. Delsuc*
Institut de Génétique et de Biologie Moléculaire
et Cellulaire (IGBMC), Illkirch cedex, France
NMRtec, Bioparc B, Illkirch, France

Abstract

Polyproline-II (PPII) helix is a very common regular pattern in proteins. It is observed in many protein structures, and is considered to be an important transient structure in Intrinsically Disordered Proteins. This structure is also part of the recognition element for the SH3 domains, which are an essential element for signal transmission into the cell.

While numerous studies and models have been made on this structure, a detailed understanding of the PPII helices behavior is still lacking. The aim of this chapter is to explore this structure by different biophysical approaches, in order to improve the PPII model available.

*E-mail address: madelsuc@unistra.fr

A series of polyproline peptides of varying lengths from 3 to 20 were studied by NMR. Hydrodynamics parameters such as diffusion coefficients were measured. These values were interpreted in terms of the fractal dimension, an hydrodynamic value evaluating the interaction between a molecule and the solvent.

This analysis confirms that the PPII helix is indeed an extended and rigid structure. However, it was shown that a minimum of 6 sequential prolines are needed and that shorter proline stretches do not display a full PPII pattern.

Moreover, diffusion coefficient measures were compared to calculations obtained by several diffusion models. It appears that most of these models, developed for the general case, are not well adapted to PPII helices and are not always able to provide results close to the experimental values. Some trends appear from this comparison nonetheless, and it is found that molecular models seem better suited to describe PPII helices than continuous models.

Finally, we generated several thousands of PPII helix conformers by varying the dihedral angles around the canonical values, as well as generating a given amount of cis prolines. This ensemble of conformers was then used as a pattern to evaluate the effect of cis-proline on the measure. All these results help creating a complete overview of PPII helices but also stress that biophysical methods would certainly be one of the best ways of studying this kind of biological patterns.

1. Introduction

Proline is a very special amino-acid. For example, it is the only one to adopt naturally cis isomers in 2 to 10% of the cases [1, 2, 3]. In spite of its unusual properties, it can be inserted in repetitive structural patterns: polyproline helices. The polyproline-I (PPI) helix is not stable in water [4] but the polyproline-II (PPII) helix is present in proteins. The latter is a left-handed helix that can be adopted by several kinds of amino-acid [5, 2, 6]. It is composed of three residues per turn and its length is about 3.2Å per amino-acid. This is the longest protein structure element ever described.

Although there is no complete explanation on its formation, which is not stabilized by hydrogen bonds, PPII helix is an important feature for signal transmission inside the cell [7, 6, 8, 9]. PPII helix is generally considered as a very rigid and extended cylinder[10]. However, models already designed to describe the behaviour of such an helix in solution tend to disagree with experimental data [11].

Having a model of this helix is necessary to understand its interaction with its protein partners. In this chapter, leads are investigated in order to develop a more comprehensive model of PPII helices, especially concerning biophysical studies.

Indeed, several biophysical parameters such as diffusion coefficients D or the fractal dimension d_f can be easily measured. d_f is a hydrodynamic parameter evaluating the interaction between a molecule and its environment which is related to the way a 3D element fills up space [12]. It can be calculated from D, which can be measured by NMR-DOSY experiments. Theoretically, for an infinite cylinder d_f = 1 and for denaturated proteins d_f = 1.71 [12]. The fractal dimension of a series of polyproline peptides was computed and compared to these theoretical values to have more information on the global shape of these peptides in solution.

Then, diffusion coefficients of this series of peptides were computed by two different methods and compared to the experimental values. Thanks to Ortega and Garcia de la Torre's equations [13], it is possible to calculate the diffusion coefficient of a cylinder of diameter d and length l as follows:

$$D = \frac{kT}{6\pi\eta(\frac{3l}{16d^2})^{\frac{1}{3}}(1.009 + 0.01395\,ln(\frac{l}{d}) + 0.0788\,ln(\frac{l}{d})^2)} \tag{1}$$

On the other hand, Marsh's equation[14] is adapted to intrinsically disordered proteins (IDP) with N residues and P percents of proline in their sequence:

$$D = \frac{kT}{6\pi\eta(2.40(1.24P + 0.904)N^{0.509})} \tag{2}$$

P is called by the authors "proline correction" as proline tends to behave differently than other amino-acids and adopts specific conformations.

Finally, a bioinformatics approach has been developed. A large number of conformers of polyproline peptides have been generated *in silico* and studied to design a new model of PPII helices.

2. Methods

2.1. Experimental Fractal Dimension

Diffusion coefficients of seven polyproline peptides (P_3, P_6, P_6C, $P_{11}C$, $P_{14}C$, $P_{20}C$) was measured by a NMR-DOSY experiment on a Bruker Avance 600MHz spectrometer equiped with a cryo-probe at 300K. Solutions were prepared with 1mM peptide, 1mM TRIS and 2eq DTT. Pulse sequence was based on stimulated echo with bipolar gradients and excitation sculpting [15]. Gradients lasted 2.8ms, 150ms were inserted between the two gradients and 5ms of *led* were necessary [16]. 40 points have been recorded with 32 scans each.

Diffusivities relative to TRIS, D_r, were computed. Fractal dimension was extracted from the slope of the linear regression done on the four biggest peptides of the $ln(D_r) = f(ln(M))$ curve.

2.2. Theoretical Fractal Dimension

Diffusion coefficients were calculated thanks to equations 1 and 2. Temperature T was settled to 300K and η to 10^{-3} Pa.s. D_r were computed thanks to the experimental values of TRIS diffusion coefficients.

2.3. Conformer Generation

Python library MMTK [17] was used to generate P_{20} conformers. A template was created to be loaded into MMTK. A large amount of conformers were created by changing randomly the dihedral angles of each amino-acid and adding the right number of cis-prolines. Conformers with steric clashes were rejected. Backbone atoms of the other conformers were then fixed and the free energy of the system was minimized in the Amber99 forcefield. Conformers containing atoms separated by less than 0.9Å were also rejected. 20 000 conformers were generated this way.

2.3.1. Fractal Dimension Calculation

Iterative computation of end-to-end distances (on the C_α), d, of parts of a conformer with n residues from an end of the conformer to the other was implemented. Fractal dimension of the conformer is the inverse of the slope of the

$ln(d) = ln(n)$ curve. These values are averaged on all conformers to give the fractal dimension of the ensemble.

2.3.2. RamaDA Analysis

Each conformer of an ensemble was analyzed by the RamaDA software [18]. Percentages of presence of each amino-acid of the peptide in the seven conformational domains defined by RamaDA were calculated and presented into a bar graph.

3. Results and Discussion

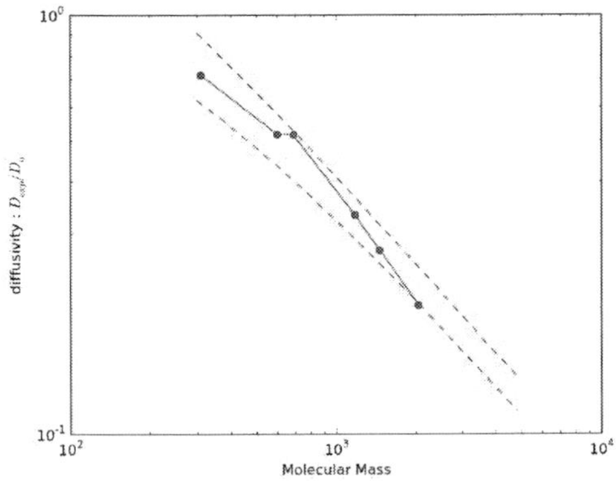

Figure 1. Diffusivity of polyproline peptides versus their molecular mass (in green). Theoretical curves computed for a cylinder from Ortega and Garcia de la Torre's equation (in red) for a length of 3.2Å per residues and diameters of 4.6Å (up) and 8.0Å (down).

Figure 1 displays the diffusion coeffients of the polyproline peptides series versus their molecular mass. The fractal dimension of this family of peptides, deduced from the diffusion coefficient values, is 1.2. This fractal dimension is lower than the lowest value observed so far on proteins, namely $d_f = 1.71$, for denaturated peptides [19, 12]. It is nonetheless really close of the fractal dimension of infinite cylinders ($d_f = 1$). It confirms that polyproline peptide adopt a rigid and very extended structure.

To validate this measure and extract its meaning, several models were used to predict the values of polyproline peptides diffusion coefficients. Ortega and Garcia de la Torre's equations (eq 1) allow the calculation of cylinders diffusion coefficients. This model can be used because the measured fractal dimension is very low so a polyproline peptide can be considered to behave as a cylinder. Results of these calculations are shown in Figure 1 for a very long cylinder (3.2Å per amino-acid) and two different cylinder diameters (4.6Å and 8.0Å). Neither of them is able to fit the measured diffusion coefficients. Either polyproline peptides oligomerize to form bigger cylinders or Ortega and Garcia de la Torre's equations are not adapted to the study of polyproline stretches.

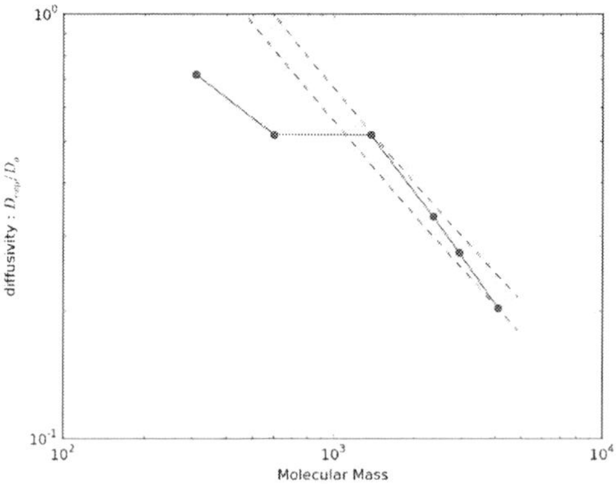

Figure 2. Diffusivity of dimerized polyproline peptides versus their molecular mass (in green). (The two lower mass points correspond to the P_3 and P_6 peptides which do not contain a terminal cystein) Theoretical curves computed for a cylinder from Ortega and Garcia de la Torre's equation (in red) for a length of 3.2Å per residues and diameters of 1.1Å (up) and 1.9Å (down).

For the peptides studied in this chapter, there are two major ways of oligomerizing. On one hand, their terminal cystein can bind another one and create a disulfide bond. On the other hand, three polyproline peptides can create a collagene helice. These two possibilities change the molecular mass of the objects observed by NMR-DOSY. Figures 2 and 3 show the results of Ortega and

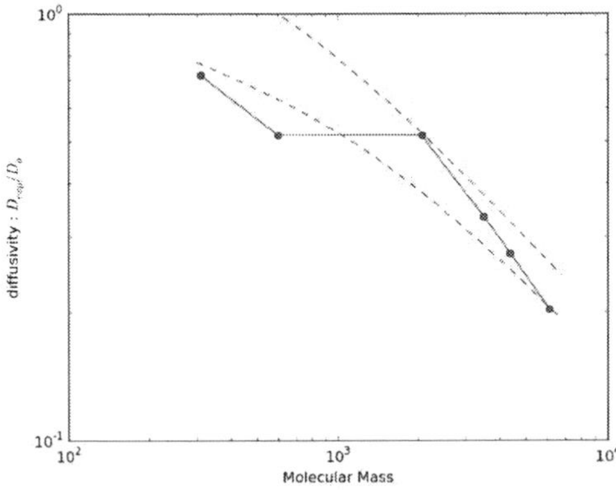

Figure 3. Diffusivity of trimerized polyproline peptides versus their molecular mass (in green). Theoretical curves computed for a cylinder from Ortega and Garcia de la Torre's equation (in red) for a length of 2.9Å per residues and diameters of 4.5Å (up) and 8.8Å (down).

Garcia de la Torre's equations for each possibility. It appears clearly that none of the experimental curve can be fitted with the equation. As a consequence, we can say that Ortega and Garcia de la Torre's equations may not be adapted to the study of polyproline peptides.

Because of these results, one can not be sure that the cylindrical model used to describe polyproline peptides is right. Nonetheless, Marsh's method (eq 2) to predict hydrodynamic radius of IDPs was designed with no assumption on proteins behaviours in solution. Thanks to this equation, it is possible to calculate theoretical values of diffusion coefficients and to compare them with the experimental ones (see figure 4). One can see that without the so-called proline correction ($P = 0$), theoretical values are close to the experimental ones. However, it appears that Marsh's equation fixes the fractal dimension to 1.96 for all the IDP, which is a very restrictive assumption and makes this equation not adapted to the study of polyproline peptides. Only P_3 and P_6 are well fitted by Marsh's equation, we may deduce that these peptides are too short to present a PPII helix form.

Actually, to our knowledge, there is no equation or method which is able to fit our data. The fractal dimension seems to be one of the best ways to recognize

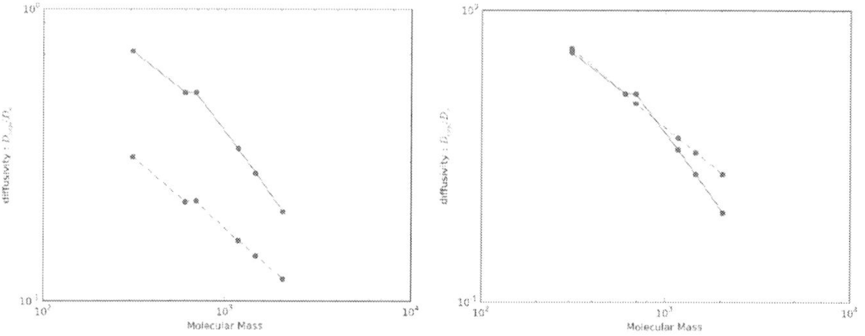

Figure 4. Comparison between diffusivity experimental values for polyproline peptides (in green) and values computed with equation 2 (in red), with (left) or without (right) proline correction.

PPII helices even though we can not describe its behaviour yet. If polyproline peptides can not be considered as cylinder, another model has to be found. On the other hand, proline is a very special amino-acid as its two isomers, cis and trans, can be appear naturally within a protein.

To assess the potential impact of such a property on the behaviour of polyproline peptides, 20 000 conformers of all-trans P_{20} were generated at first. Figure 5 shows the average C_α-C_α distances matrix and a RamaDA analysis of this ensemble. From the C_α-C_α matrix, it seems that no particular structure can be observed in the P_{20} peptides. However, when one look closely to the proportion of conformers given by RamaDA, it is clear that P_{20} displays PPII helices, as expected. The fractal dimension calculated on this ensemble $d_f = 1.12$ is very close to the experimental value.

Three other ensembles were generated with respectively 2%, 5% and 10% of cis-prolines randomly placed along the polyproline chain. Figure 6 and table 1 compare the results for the four ensembles. C_α-C_α matrices and R_g calculations show that the higher the percentage of cis-prolines, the more compact the peptide is. What is really striking is the fact that it is possible to find the experimental value of fractal dimension for a percentage of cis-prolines between 2 and 5%. This value agrees with previous studies on cis-prolines.

Then, a new model of polyproline peptides can be designed. Polyproline peptides may behave not as one cylinder but as several cylinders linked by cis-

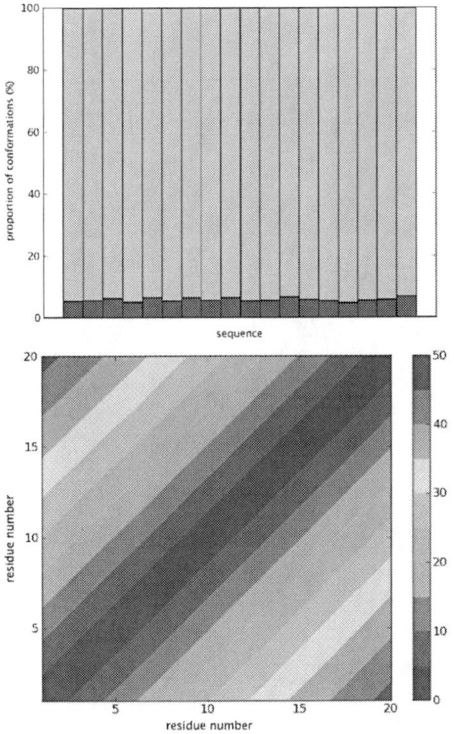

Figure 5. RamaDA analysis of conformers ensemble (top, in yellow the proportions of PPII conformations and in blue helical conformations) and Cα-Cα distances matrix (bottom).

Table 1. Values of fractal dimension and average radius of gyration depending on the proportion of cis-proline in conformer ensembles

Pourcentage de cis-prolines	d_f	R_g (Å)
0%	1.12	15.78 ± 1.60
2%	1.16	15.06 ± 2.01
5%	1.22	14.04 ± 2.36
10%	1.31	12.79 ± 2.45

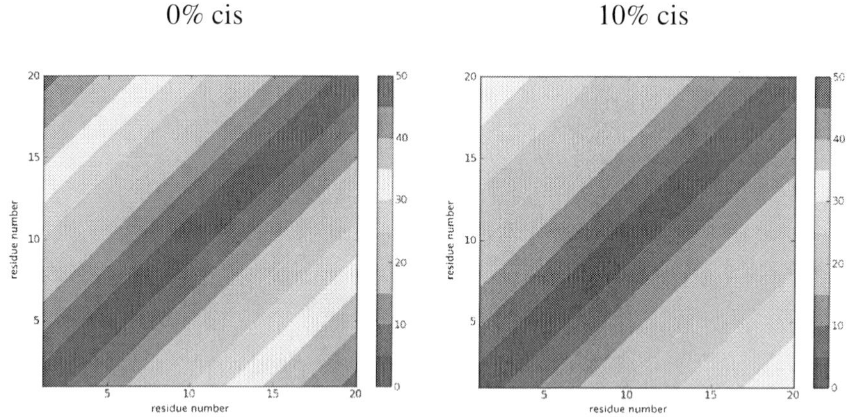

Figure 6. $C\alpha$-$C\alpha$ distances matrices for conformer ensembles with 0% (left) and 10% (right) cis-prolines.

prolines.

4. Conclusion

The fractal dimension computed for a series of polyproline peptides is 1.2, which is really close to the fractal dimension of an infinite cylinder. This value confirms that PPII helices are very extended and rather rigid.

However, PPII helices can not be considered as cylinders because Ortega and Gracia de la Torre's equation results do not fit the experimental data. Moreover, Marsh's equation can not be used as well because it considers that IDPs always have the same d_f,which is not the case.

Another model has to be developed to understand the behaviour of PPII helices. In this purpose, 20 000 conformers of a polyproline peptide, P_{20}, were generated *in silico* to gather a maximum of information. By analysing the impact of the cis-trans isomerism of prolines, it appears that the experimental fractal dimension can be explained by 2 to 5% of cis-prolines.

Thanks to all these studies, it is possible to design a new model. Indeed, polyproline peptides may be considered not as one long cylinder but as several cylinders linked by cis-prolines.

This model needs to be validated by other experiments but is already useful to understand the fractal dimension of the peptides, which can not be explained by any of the other models tested.

References

[1] Best RB, Merchant KA, Gopich IV, Schuler B, Bax A, Eaton WA: Effect of flexibility and cis residues in single-molecule FRET studies of polyproline. *Proc Natl Acad Sci USA* 2007, 104(48):18964–9.

[2] Vila J, Baldoni H, Ripoll D, Ghosh A, Scheraga H: Polyproline II helix conformation in a proline-rich environment: A theoretical study. *Biophys J* 2004, 86(2):731–742.

[3] Dolghih E, Ortiz W, Kim S, Krueger BP, Krause JL, Roitberg AE: Theoretical Studies of Short Polyproline Systems: Recalibration of a Molecular Ruler. *J Phys Chem A* 2009, 113(16):4639–4646.

[4] Kakinoki S, Hirano Y, Oka M: On the stability of polyproline-I and II structures of proline oligopeptides. *Polym Bull* 2005, 53(2):109–115.

[5] Kelly MA, Chellgren BW, Rucker AL, Troutman JM, Fried MG, Miller AF, Creamer TP: Host-guest study of left-handed polyproline II helix formation. *Biochemistry* 2001, 40(48):14376–83.

[6] Cubellis MV, Caillez F, Blundell TL, Lovell SC: Properties of polyproline II, a secondary structure element implicated in protein-protein interactions. *Proteins* 2005, 58(4):880–92.

[7] Rath A, Davidson AR, Deber CM: The structure of "unstructured" regions in peptides and proteins: role of the polyproline II helix in protein folding and recognition. *Biopolymers* 2005, 80(2-3):179–85.

[8] Mayer BJ: SH3 domains: complexity in moderation. *J Cell Sci* 2001, 114(Pt 7):1253–63.

[9] Bour G, Gaillard E, Bruck N, Lalevée S, Plassat JL, Busso D, Samama JP, Rochette-Egly C: Cyclin H binding to the RARalpha activation function (AF)-2 domain directs phosphorylation of the AF-1 domain by cyclin-dependent kinase 7. *Proc Natl Acad Sci USA* 2005, 102(46):16608–13.

[10] Stryer L, Haugland RP: Energy transfer: a spectroscopic ruler. *Proc Natl Acad Sci USA* 1967, 58(2):719–26.

[11] Doose S, Neuweiler H, Barsch H, Sauer M: Probing polyproline structure and dynamics by photoinduced electron transfer provides evidence for deviations from a regular polyproline type II helix. *Proc Natl Acad Sci USA* 2007, 104(44):17400–5.

[12] Augé S, Schmit PO, Crutchfield CA, Islam MT, Harris DJ, Durand E, Clemancey M, Quoineaud AA, Lancelin JM, Prigent Y, Taulelle F, Delsuc MA: NMR measure of translational diffusion and fractal dimension. Application to molecular mass measurement. *J Phys Chem B* 2009, 113(7):1914–8.

[13] Ortega A, de la Torre J: Hydrodynamic properties of rodlike and disklike particles in dilute solution. *J Chem Phys* 2003, 119(18):9914–9919.

[14] Marsh JA, Forman-Kay JD: Sequence Determinants of Compaction in Intrinsically Disordered Proteins. *Biophys J* 2010, 98(10):2383–2390.

[15] Balayssac S, Delsuc MA, Gilard V, Prigent Y, Malet-Martino M: Two-dimensional DOSY experiment with Excitation Sculpting water suppression for the analysis of natural and biological media. *J Magn Reson* 2009, 196:78–83.

[16] Gibbs S, Johnson C: A PFG NMR experiment for accurate diffusion and flow studies in the presence of Eddy currents. *J Magn Reson* 1991. [Exprience LED DOSY].

[17] Hinsen K: The molecular modeling toolkit: A new approach to molecular simulations. *J Comput Chem* 2000, 21(2):79–85.

[18] Tanty M, Delsuc MA: *RamaDA: complete and automated conformational overview of proteins*. arXiv 2011, q-bio.BM. [7 pages, 3 figures, 3 tables].

[19] Wilkins DK, Grimshaw SB, Receveur V, Dobson CM, Jones JA, Smith LJ: Hydrodynamic radii of native and denatured proteins measured by pulse field gradient NMR techniques. *Biochemistry* 1999, 38(50):16424–31.

In: Proline
Editor: Bouzid Nedjimi

ISBN: 978-1-62257-739-2

Chapter V

Free Energies, Structural Characteristics and Transition Mechanisms of Proline-rich Peptides

Mahmoud Moradi, Volodymyr Babin, Christopher Roland and Celeste Sagui*

Center for High Performance Simulations (CHiPS) and Department of Physics, North Carolina State University, Raleigh, NC, US

Abstract

In this chapter, we are interested in relatively small proline-rich peptides that in spite of their apparent simplicity have generated considerable controversy in the literature. First, we explore issues related to the conformational space of pure polyproline (PP) peptides. PP peptides are

*E-mail address: sagui@ncsu.edu

generally associated with two well-characterized helical structures: (a) a left-handed polyproline helix (PPII), with all peptide bonds in the trans-isomer conformation; and (b) a more compact right-handed polyproline helix (PPI), with all the peptide bonds in the cis-isomer conformation. Because of their relatively rigid structure, PPII peptides have been used as a "molecular ruler" in structural biology, especially for the validation of spectroscopic rulers in Föster resonance energy transfer. However, recent experimental and theoretical studies have called this traditional picture of polyproline peptides as a "rigid rod" into question, since PP peptides in aqueous solution display static structural heterogeneity with subpopulations of different end-to-end distances that do not interconvert on the time scales of nano- to milliseconds. Second, we investigate the properties of guest amino acids in host proline peptides. Experimentally, there has been considerable emphasis on deriving an "intrinsic PPII propensity" scale for amino acids in a proline-rich host-guest environment, in order to understand the role of PPII conformations in denatured proteins. In particular, Circular Dichroism (CD) experiments attribute a high PPII propensity to several amino acids, a claim that has been disputed by theoretical work. In order to probe these issues, we have used classical molecular dynamics (MD) simulations, with state-of-the-art force fields and novel sampling methodology to study the free energy landscapes, conformational characteristics and equilibrium populations of pure PP peptides of various lengths in different environments and of proline-based oligopeptides with single and multiple guest amino acids. Our results point to the presence of many free energy minima associated with stable or metastable PP structures, which are characterized in terms of the cis/trans pattern of the prolyl bonds. We have also characterized several mechanisms for the interconversion between PPI and PPII structures. For the host-guest systems, we find no evidence for an intrinsic PPII propensity in any of the guest amino acids other than proline. Instead, the PPII content as derived from experiments may be explained in terms of: (i) a local correlation between the dihedral angles of the guest amino acid and the proline residue immediately preceding it; and (ii) a non-local correlation between the cis/trans states of the peptide bonds. In terms of the latter, we find that the presence of a guest (other than proline, tyrosine or tryptophan) increases the trans content of most of the prolyl bonds, which results in an effective increase of the peptide PPII content.

PACS: 05.45-a, 52.35.Mw, 96.50.Fm

Keywords: Free energy, molecular dynamics, proline-rich peptides

1. Introduction

The unique properties of the proline amino acid, including its side chain cyclized to its backbone (that restricts its backbone dihedral angle ϕ to about $-75°$), and the ability of its prolyl bond to take both $trans$- and cis-isomers make proline quite an "idiosyncratic" amino acid in the protein world. The left-handed PPII structure associated with the trans isomers plays an important role in cell processes such as transcription, signal transduction and cell motility. Proline's propensity to form left-handed helices is also crucial for cellular structural integrity, in particular for plant cell wall proteins and collagen. In collagen, three left-handed helices are twisted together into a right-handed coil, or triple helix. Here, prolines or hydroxyprolines constitute about one sixth of the total sequence (with glycine contributing about one third of the sequence). PPII helices also commonly occur in globular proteins [1], where the tendency of proline to stabilize PPII structures plays a crucial role in ligands of the protein domains such as WW and EVH1. The SH3 (Src homology 3) domains have been shown to mediate protein-protein interactions by binding to Pro-rich sequences of 10 amino acids in a PPII conformation [2, 3]. The requirement that the Pro-rich ligands be in a PPII conformation is also of interest because such conformations can have therapeutic applications, since SH3 domains are found in kinases, adapter proteins, lipases, GTPases, etc. Perhaps because of their important role, prolines are consistently conserved at a level of 100-80 $\%$ in proteins with a sequence identity above 20$\%$ [4]. Although not necessarily part of a PPII helix, approximately 10$\%$ of all residues are individually found in PPII conformations.

In our work, we are interested in relatively small proline-rich peptides that in spite of their apparent simplicity have generated considerable controversy in the literature[5, 6, 7, 8, 9]. The challenges in the study of these peptides relates directly to the nature of the proline amino acid and the correlations it generates in the presence of other amino acids. First, we explore issues related to the conformational space of polyproline (PP) peptides. Traditionally, it is believed that the rigidity of these peptides, associated will all $trans$ structures, makes them useful as "molecular rulers". Second, we weigh in in the controversy related to the extent of PPII content in the denatured states of proteins.

With respect to the conformational space of PP peptides, it is helpful to review the two ideal structures of polyproline. Polyproline is known to form helical structures (see Figure 1) with two well-characterized conformations: (a) a left-handed polyproline helix (PPII) forms when all the sequential residues adopt backbone dihedral angles (ϕ, ψ) of $(-75°, 146°)$ with all prolyl bonds in the $trans$-isomer conformation (*i.e.* backbone dihedral angle $\omega = 180°$) with 3 residues per turn; and (b) a more compact right-handed polyproline helix (PPI) that forms when all sequential residues adopt dihedral angles of roughly $(-75°, 160°)$ and all prolyl bonds assume a cis-isomer conformation (*i.e.* backbone dihedral angle $\omega = 0°$) with 3.3 residues per turn.

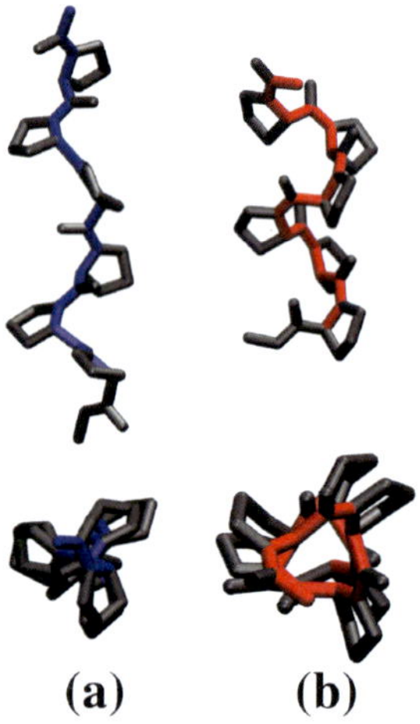

Figure 1. Side and top views of two helical conformations of a polyproline hexamer (ACE-(Pro)$_6$-NME): (a) Polyproline II helix (PPII, poly-pro II), a left-handed helix with backbone dihedral angles of $(-75°, 146°, 180°)$, respectively. (b) Polyproline I helix (PPI), a right-handed helix with backbone dihedral angles of $(\phi, \psi, \omega) = (-75°, 160°, 0°)$; trans(cis) prolyl bonds are colored blue(red).

Traditionally, the relatively rigid structure of PPII has been used as a "molecular ruler" in structural biology, especially for the validation of spectroscopic rulers in Föster resonance energy transfer (FRET) experiments [10]. However, recent studies have put the traditional picture of polyproline peptide as a rigid rod with all-$trans$ proline residues and randomly rotating dyes attached by defined spacers [11, 12, 13, 14, 15, 16, 17, 5] in question. Both FRET and photoinduced-electron transfer (PET) studies show deviations in the experimentally observed end-to-end distances of polyproline from its theoretical predictions. Doose *et* al. used PET techniques to probe the structure and dynamics of PPII with 1-10 residues in an aqueous solution [16], and showed that "polyproline samples exhibit static structural heterogeneity with subpopulations having distinct end-to-end distances that do not interconvert on the scales from nano- to milliseconds". This heterogeneity was attributed to interspersed cis isomers that disrupt the otherwise ideal all-trans PPII structure, in agreement with theoretical studies based on conformational energy calculations[18] and previous simulation results [19]. The authors concluded that the stability of these heterogeneous subpopulations, caused by prolyl cis/trans isomerization, requires characterization of the cis isomers in order for polyproline to be used as a molecular ruler, *i.e.*, in order to calibrate FRET efficiency measurements. Clearly, the probability distribution of cis/trans prolyl bonds will be affected by neighboring amino acids [20, 21], pH and ionic strength [22], solvent [23, 24, 25, 26, 27, 28, 29] and chain length[30]. For the most part, it has been noted experimentally that the left-handed PPII structure is favored in water, benzyl alcohol, trifluoroethanol, organic acids, and most of the other solvents, while the PPI structure is favored in the presence of aliphatic alcohols like propanol [31, 32, 33, 30].

PPII helices are also believed to play an important role in the denatured states of proteins, even for molecules that do not contain a single proline, such as diverse Ala-based peptides. Initially, the left-handed PPII conformation was proposed as an alternate to the random coil model for disordered peptides and unfolded proteins by Tiffany and Krimm in 1968 [34]. This hypothesis arose from the experimentally observed similarities between the ultraviolet circular dichroism (CD) spectra of denatured proteins and that of PPII [35]. This proposition was revived in the last ten years with a common consensus, that, indeed PPII conformations are part of the denatured states. However, there is considerable dissent with regards to the proportion of these PPII states versus other states. Thus, for Ala-rich peptides, the two contrasting views are that Ala has a very high PPII propensity (between 80% and 100%) [36, 37, 38, 39, 40, 41, 42, 43]; or that the PPII conformation is just one of many local conformational states, and not the overall conformation of the unfolded peptides [44, 45, 46, 47, 19, 48, 49, 50, 51, 52, 53].

Experimentally, there has been considerable emphasis on deriving an intrinsic PPII propensity scale for individual amino acids in a proline-rich host-guest environment [54, 55, 56, 57, 58, 59, 60]. This scale is based on host-guest experiments, which is a powerful tool for probing the overall structural characteristics of peptides, such as their α-helix [61, 62] and β-sheets [63, 64] content. In the proline-based experiments, a guest residue, X is inserted in a short polyproline peptide of the form Ace$-$(Pro)$_3$$-X-(Pro)_3$$-Gly-Tyr-NH_2$, termed PXP for brevity. Since a proline guest (X=P) is expected to form a stable PPII helix in aqueous solution, deviations from this conformation induced by non-proline guests are expected to provide a measure of their PPII propensity. In particular, the CD spectrum of PPP at 5°C possesses a minimum at 205 nm and a maximum at 228 nm [55, 56]. A significantly smaller molar ellipticity is a sign of shorter helices and/or less PPII helical content [65]. Since disordered peptides and proteins also possess a minimum in this region of the spectrum, this minimum makes a poor choice for characterization of the PPII helical content. Instead, the PPII helical content has been estimated to vary linearly with the maximum molar ellipticity at 228 nm. With Circular Dichroism (CD) experiments, it was found that the presence of non-proline guests decreases the PPII helical content, although the range of PPII helical content is relatively narrow. This is a consequence of the host peptide design, which forces at least four prolines to be in the PPII conformation. The PPP peptide was found, on average, to be 67% PPII helical, and other amino acids such as Gln, Ala and Gly were deemed to have high PPII propensity in this context [55, 56, 57]. In addition, peptides with two guest Ala's were also investigated, *i.e.*, Ace$-$(Pro)$_3-$(Ala)$_2-$(Pro)$_3-$Gly$-$Tyr$-NH_2$ (PAAP for short). The studies concluded that PAAP also possesses a high PPII content, and that the PPII helix can propagate through two adjacent non-proline residues[55]. It was further proposed that PPII is the energetically most favorable conformation, because all backbone polar groups are solvated in water which compensates for the lack of intramolecular hydrogen bonds. The assumption here is that all the proline residues should be in their trans conformation, since in the cis conformation the carboxyl oxygen atoms tend to lie parallel to the backbone hidden from the water. These studies were taken as further proof that Ala has a relatively high PPII propensity, based on the following rationale. While a proline can restrict its preceding residue through steric interactions[66], the Ala guest was deemed not to have much effect in the preceding proline. This unconstrained proline was expected to adopt all accessible conformations, thus decreasing the PPII content considerably below that measured for PAP, unless Ala itself contributed to this content by means of an "intrinsic" PPII propensity.

Subsequently, Vila *et al.*[19] investigated this problem theoretically, obtaining PPII contents for the different host-guest peptides in qualitative agreement with the experimental numbers. Specifically, they noted a reduction in the PPII helical content with respect to the PPP peptide. By mapping the lowest energy conformations into the Zimmerman regions of the Ramachandran plot, the authors concluded that there is no propagation of the PPII conformational preference into the guest for the PXP residues they analyzed (X= Ala, Gln, Gly, Val) for the simple reason that none of these residues is found in the F region of the map. Furthermore, the notion that a solvated proline-rich peptide take on its optimal conformation only was deemed to be an oversimplification. Instead, the dynamical changes associated with the cis/trans isomerization of the proline residues[19] need to be accounted for, and that the notion of an "intrinsic PPII propensity" would need revision.

Intrigued by these studies and the on-going debate concerning both the conformational characteristics of pure proline oligomers and the intrinsic PPII propensity of non-proline amino acids, we have re-examined these problems using new free energy methods in combination with classical molecular dynamics with state-of-the-art force fields to study the structural characteristics of proline-based oligopeptides with and without guest amino acids [5, 6, 7, 8, 9]. Specifically, we have characterized the conformational preferences associated with the cis/trans isomerization of the prolyl bonds, the puckering of the pyrrolidine rings, and the secondary structural motifs associated with the dihedral angles of the Ramachandran plots of the different proline and/or non-proline residues of several short polyproline and proline-rich peptides.

From a computational point of view, the characterization of the proline-based structures is rather difficult, since the cis/trans isomerization is much slower than the formation and rupture of hydrogen bonds in an α helix-coil transition. Indeed, characteristic time scales for prolyl isomerization range in tens to hundreds of seconds at room temperature [67, 20], indicating an energy barrier of the order of 10 to 20 kcal/mol [68, 69, 70, 71, 72, 73, 74]. Due to these huge energy barriers, traditional molecular dynamics (MD) simulations cannot explore the relevant conformational space. Hence, we made use of several complementary free energy methods, including the Adaptively Biased Molecular Dynamics (ABMD) [75], Replica-Exchange Molecular Dynamics (REMD), and Steered Molecular Dynamics (SMD). In particular, ABMD was used to compute the free energy surface of a set of collective variables; REMD was used to improve the performance of ABMD and to facilitate the sampling of equilibrium configurations directly; and SMD was used to study different transition mechanisms directly.

This Chapter is organized as follows. The free energy methodology, collective variables and analysis used is discussed in the next Section. Section 3 presents a review of our recent work with regards to pure polyproline peptides [5, 6, 7] including free energies, structural characteristics, and PPI-PPII transition mechanisms in different solvent environments. Section 4 reviews our recent work regarding the host-guest peptides [8, 9] for single and multiple guests. Finally, the last Section is reserved for a summary of the key results.

2. Methodology

Classical molecular dynamics (MD) is a powerful computational technique to study the atomistic details of biomolecular phenomena, particularly when the experimental techniques cannot provide a detailed dynamical description of the phenomena. However, due to the computational limitations, typical room-temperature MD is incapable of generating the complete conformational distributions associated with the so-called "slow modes" of the system that require crossing high free energy barriers. Fortunately, new advances in sampling techniques – particularly over the last decade – have enabled MD to overcome some of these issues. MD combined with novel enhanced sampling techniques can be used to accurately (within a given model) calculate the free energies and other relevant characteristics of biomolecular systems.

In this Section, we review the complementary free energy techniques used in our investigations, *i.e.*, the ABMD [75], SMD [76], and REMD [77] methodology. Our discussion will be quite brief since these methods, along with any relevant simulation details, have been extensively documented in the literature [5, 6, 7, 8, 9]. In addition, in order to understand our results, we define the so-called "collective variables" used in our investigations. Finally, we provide details of our simulation analysis including the calculation of secondary structural motifs of peptides, details on how to quantify the PPII content of a peptide, as well as a review of the Odds Ratio construction as a useful analytical tool for inferring the statistical influence of secondary structures.

2.1. Free Energy Methods and Enhanced Sampling

The free energy is the key quantity for the prediction of the delicate *three-dimensional* structure of biomolecules, their binding, the chemical reactions they catalyze, the molecular recognition problem, and –on a larger length scale– the balance between different biological systems. Typical biomolecular free energy surfaces (FES) are quite rugged and complex, and therefore very long times are needed in order to fully explore a given FES. This is generally precluded in a regular MD simulation. Over the past few years, several methods targeting the computation of the free energy using non-equilibrium simulations have become popular. These include the Local Elevation Method [78], the adaptive-force bias method [79], the Wang-Landau approach [80], and the metadynamics method [81, 82]. These methods all provide for an elegant way of computing the Landau free energy or potential of mean force (PMF) as a function of a collective variable $\sigma(\mathbf{r}_1, \ldots, \mathbf{r}_N)$ from an "evolving" ensemble of realizations [83, 84], and use that estimate to bias the system dynamics so as to flatten the effective free energy surface. The collective variables provide for a reduced dimensionality description of the system, with the rest of degrees of freedom integrated out. The free energy is then given via:

$$f(\xi) = -k_B T \ln p(\xi),$$

where k_B is the Boltzmann constant, T is the temperature, and $p(\xi) = \langle \delta \left[\xi - \sigma(\mathbf{r}_1, \ldots, \mathbf{r}_N) \right] \rangle$ is the equilibrium probability density of the collective variable (the angular brackets denote an ensemble average). Collectively, these methods may all be considered as umbrella sampling methods with an evolving potential.

Our calculation of accurate free energies is based on the ABMD method [75] complemented with SMD simulations [76] as integrated in the AMBER software package [85]. Although spatial constraints make it difficult to review the technical aspects of the ABMD method here, there are two important extensions associated with our implementation that are worth commenting on. Both of these lead to a more uniform flattening of the effective free energy surface due to an improved sampling of the evolving canonical distribution. The first extension is identical in spirit to the multiple walkers metadynamics [83, 86]. It amounts to carrying out several different MD simulations biased by the same effective potential, which is "flattened" by all these walkers simultaneously. A second extension is to gather several different MD trajectories, each bearing its own biasing potential and, if desired, its own temperature and/or collective variables, into a generalized ensemble for *replica exchange* with modified exchange rules [87, 84]. We also allow for either an evolving, or a static, biasing potential. When all biasing potentials are static, the method reduces to a variant of the "Hamiltonian Replica Exchange" method [87]. Exchanges between random pairs of replicas are attempted at a prescribed rate. This procedure ultimately can yield highly accurate free energies, and has already been applied to a variety of different biomolecular systems including the short β-hairpin peptide [88, 75, 89], sugar puckering [90], polyproline systems [5, 6, 7, 8, 9], DNA, and

α-helix forming systems.

As a complement to the ABMD method, we use SMD simulations to examine transition pathways and mechanisms, as well as to estimate free energy differences [6, 7]. The SMD method is based on the following ideas. Consider a thermodynamic process that changes a system by means of a control parameter ξ, which runs from ξ_0 to ξ_t over a time interval t. The second law of thermodynamics states that the work W done on the system cannot be smaller than the free energy difference: $\Delta F = f(\xi_t) - f(\xi_0) \leq W$. Thus, a nonequilibrium process can only provide us with an upper bound for the free energy difference. However, the remarkable Jarzynski[91] equality (JE),

$$\exp(-\Delta F/k_B T) = \langle \exp(-W/k_B T) \rangle,$$

holds even when the transformation is irreversible (the angular brackets denote the average over all possible realizations of the process connecting the states ξ_0 and ξ_t). Thus, in principle ΔF can be estimated using a number of finite-time *nonequilibrium* simulations. Unfortunately, because the average of the exponential function is dominated by rare realizations, convergence is often poor unless a very large number of runs is used. It is, however, possible to improve the free energy estimates by using modifications based on the maximum likelihood estimator (MLE) and Bennet's acceptance ratio (BAR) method, which are considered to be equivalent [92, 93, 94]. These methods make use of both forward and reverse non-equilibrium pulling processes, in order to take the system from an initial to a final state. Typically, the system is moved along a specific pathway in its configurational space, which is readily accomplished through the addition of a harmonic restraining potential to the Hamiltonian in the stiff-spring limit [6]. We have used SMD to move various system between different states over the ABMD FES, thereby probing different transition mechanisms and their associated barriers, and estimating free energy differences. It comes as no surprise that the modified formula based on BAR methods shows the fastest convergence and best results [6].

Although the free energy maps can be used to characterize the properties of a system in terms of one or more collective variables, it is often desirable to sample unbiased equilibrium configurations directly. In this case, the approximate free energies computed via ABMD may be used to set up the Hamiltonian Replica Exchange Molecular Dynamics (HREMD) simulations for enhanced equilibrium sampling[90]. Typically, several replicas running at the lowest temperature T_0, are introduced into the setup. One of the replicas is completely unbiased, and therefore samples the unbiased Boltzmann distribution at $T = T_0$. The other replicas are subject to a reduced bias at T_0. These "proxy" replicas ensure adequate exchange rates and hence enhance the mixing.

In the most general case, the barrier crossings are enhanced in different replicas by means of a temperature ladder and/or biasing potentials: the former is not specific to any particular feature of the system, while the latter allows for an accentuation of some modes (for example, cis/trans transitions of the prolyl bonds for the polyproline system to be discussed later). In many cases both devices may be necessary for robust REMD simulations. The ergodic time scale of a REMD simulation is largely determined by two factors: the efficiency of the random walk between the replicas, and the fastest ergodic time scale present among the individual replicas. The first factor can be described in terms of the exchange rates between the pairs of replicas and, as long as the rates are sufficiently high, need not be considered. The replica characterized by the fastest ergodic time scale is usually referred to as the "hottest" one. Typically, it is the replica running at the highest temperature. Its mixing properties can be assessed by simulating it alone, making sure that it is ergodic, and that its autocorrelation time is sufficiently small so as to generate enough independent samples in a feasible runtime. In a practical setting, the number of replicas is typically limited and hence the "hottest" replica must be constructed with care. In principle it is always possible to use just the temperature alone (however, the higher the temperature of the "hottest" replica, the more replicas are needed to span the temperatures down to lowest T_0), or to use the biasing potentials alone (running all the replicas at the same temperature). The second scenario is not always practical, as it is considerably less generic than the first one. A combination of Hamiltonian and Temperature REMD methods (HT-REMD[95, 6]) could provide a practical way to reduce the computational costs of the REMD sampling, as it permits one to facilitate the sampling in the "hottest" replica by using both means thus allowing for better "tuning" of the entire setup.

2.1.1. Collective Variables

Methods such as ABMD calculate the free energy landscapes as a function of *one* or *two* collective variables. Higher-dimensional free energy maps are typically impractical due to the associated computational costs. Free energy maps, obtained from ABMD simulations can also be used in a H-REMD or HT-REMD setting to produce large conformational ensembles. Collective variables are also necessary in the SMD protocols. In all these cases, the collective variables were chosen to reflect the "slow modes" of the system. For proline-based peptides, these are primarily associated with the *cis/trans* isomerization of the prolyl bonds. The "fast modes", characterized by changes on relatively short time scales, are properly sampled and therefore *de facto* integrated out when calculating the Landau free energy. For instance, an important example of a fast mode is provided by the puckering of the pyrrolidine ring that is known to adopt distinct up- and down-puckered conformations[96] deemed initially to be almost equally probable[97, 98]. The solvated transition barrier between the puckered up and down states of the system is of the order of a few $k_B T$[99, 5]. At room temperature, the ring therefore rapidly oscillates between its two states, so that the puckering effects are effectively integrated out when the ensemble averages are calculated[5, 7]. The collective variables used in this study are based on criteria of peptide handedness, length and the cis/trans isomerization of the peptide bonds.

Since the peptides form chiral helices, a collective variable involving handedness (H) is natural to contemplate. To define such a collective variable [5], a sequence of four points A, B, C, , D along a given helix is chosen. These points determine the vectors $\overrightarrow{AB}$ and $\overrightarrow{CD}$. The midpoints of these vectors (E and F) form the vector $\overrightarrow{EF}$. The handedness of these points is then defined as:

$$H_{ABCD} = \frac{\overrightarrow{EF} \cdot \overrightarrow{CD} \times \overrightarrow{AB}}{|\overrightarrow{EF}|.|\overrightarrow{CD}|.|\overrightarrow{AB}|}, \tag{1}$$

Such a definition discriminates between right-handed ($H_{ABCD} > 0$) helices and left-handed ($H_{ABCD} < 0$) helices. To complete the definition, the four-point contributions are then summed along the backbone, thereby defining the collective variable H for the entire peptide: $H = \sum_{i=1}^{n-3} H_{i,i+1,i+2,i+3}$, Roughly speaking, the magnitude of H is a measure of the number of turns associated with the helices. For polyproline, the position of the nitrogen atoms was found to be a good choice for the location of the $A, \ldots, D$ points.

Even though the handedness is enough to differentiate between PPI and PPII, many compact structures are characterized by the same value of H. To remove this degeneracy, we considered the free energies associated with the radius of gyration R_g of the heavy atoms: $R_g = \sqrt{\sum_a \frac{m_a}{m_\Sigma} (\mathbf{r}_a - \mathbf{R}_\Sigma)^2}$. Here, $\mathbf{R}_\Sigma = \sum_a (m_a/m_\Sigma)\, \mathbf{r}_a$ is the center of mass; $m_\Sigma = \sum_a m_a$, and the sums run over all atoms except hydrogen. Note that R_g is not the only quantity that can be used to characterize the spatial extent of a peptide's conformation. Experimentally, results are often discussed in terms of the end-to-end distance (d_{end}), which provided equivalent information to R_g about the peptide length [5].

For the polyproline peptides, the most useful collective variables are associated with the $cis/trans$ isomerization, *i.e.*, the change that the torsion angle makes from cis (C) ($\omega = 0°$) to $trans$ (T) ($\omega = 180°$). This allows for the definition of new, convenient collective variables. For instance, we define Ω as the sum of the cosines of the ω angles, which for an n-mer polyproline peptide with $n-1$ prolyl bonds is:

$$\Omega_{n-mer} = \sum_{i=1}^{n-1} \cos \omega_i. \tag{2}$$

For a C (T) prolyl bond, $\cos \omega_i$ is $+1$ (-1) and therefore Ω_{n-mer} can take any of the following values: $-n+1$, $-n+3$, . . ., $n-3$, or $n-1$. This collective variable Ω gives the net balance of C and T prolyl bonds and obviously has some degeneracy. For a sequence with $n_b = n-1$ bonds where each bond can be in either C or T, the number of conformations with n_C C bonds and n_T T bonds (with $n_b = n_C + n_T$) is $n_b!/(n_C!n_T!)$. Naturally, perfect PPI is characterized by $\Omega_{n-mer} = n-1$ and perfect PPII by $\Omega_{n-mer} = -(n-1)$.

Alternatively, one can consider the "interface" between bonds, and define a collective variable Λ as:

$$\Lambda_{n-mer} = \sum_{i=1}^{n-2} \cos(\omega_i + \omega_{i+1}). \tag{3}$$

For an n-mer, there are $n-1$ prolyl bonds and $n-2$ interfaces. If two neighboring bonds have the same dihedral angle ω then their interface is $\cos(\omega_i + \omega_{i+1}) = +1$, otherwise it is -1. Correspondingly, Λ_{n-mer} can take on any of the values $-n+2$, $-n+4$, . . ., $n-4$, $n-2$. Λ_{n-mer} removes some of the degeneracy associated with Ω. For $|\Omega| = n-1$, there is only one value of Λ ($\Lambda = n-2$); for $\Omega = 0$ (that exists only for odd values of n) there are $(n-2)$ values of Λ ; for $|\Omega| = m$ (with $m \neq n-1$ and $m \neq 0$), there are $n-1-m$ values of Λ. Thus a typical free energy landscape in the (Ω, Λ) plane has a triangular shape.

Having the binary nature of dihedral angle ω, one can define many different ω-based collective variables such as Ω and Λ to identify different cis/trans patterns [6]. We note that all these dihedral angle ω-based collective variables can be generalized to any proline-containing peptide. Particularly, $\Omega = \sum_b \cos \omega_b$ (here sum runs over all the prolyl bonds) is a practical collective variable to "capture" different patterns of the cis/trans conformations in any proline-containing peptide. Particularly in the proline-rich peptides, Ω describes the slowest mode of the system.

2.2. Quantifying the PPII Propensity

To examine the concept of "intrinsic" PPII propensity of amino acids, one needs to (i) quantify the PPII content of amino acids in a system and (ii) distinguish between the intrinsic and non-intrinsic portion of this content. The latter requires an appropriate correlation analysis and the former requires not only a clear definition for the PPII secondary structure but also a practical statistical technique to measure the PPII content from a large conformational ensemble.

2.2.1. Identifying Secondary Structures

We used the (ϕ, ψ) dihedral angles to identify different regions [100] of the Ramachandran map [101]. According to this scheme, the α region is divided into two parts: α_R defined by $-120° < \psi < 90°$ and $-160° < \phi < -20°$ and α_L defined by $-50° < \psi < 110°$ and $20° < \phi < 160°$. The F region includes $-110° < \phi < -20°$ and $(90° < \psi < 180°$ or $-180° < \psi < -120°)$. The β region consists of two parts: $(-180° < \phi < -110°, 90° < \psi < 180°$ or $-180° < \psi < -120°)$ and $(160° < \phi < 180°$ and $120° < \psi < 180°)$ regions.

Although this delineates clear regions for the dihedrals of most residues, it turns out that there is considerable overlap between the populations of the F and β regions. In some cases the α_R region may overlap with both the F and β regions as well. In order to handle this situation, we used a clustering technique to identify the region of the conformations, rather than strictly enforcing the sharp boundaries of a given region[102, 103]. These two methods give identical answers for most dihedrals. However, at the borders, the clustering technique is deemed to be more accurate.

For non-proline amino acids, the PPII content is simply given by its F population, because the peptide bonds are all T. However, for proline both the C and T isomers fall in the F region. Since the C isomer is a signature of the PPI structure, these were not counted here since we were interested in the PPII content of the peptide *only*. Since an ideal PPII proline residue is in a trans conformation and also in the F region, one can find the probability of each residue being in be used to characterize the spatial extent of a peptide's conformation. Experimentally, results are often discussed in terms of the end-to-end distance (d_{end}), which provided equivalent information to R_g about the peptide length [5].

For the polyproline peptides, the most useful collective variables are associated with the $cis/trans$ isomerization, *i.e.*, the change that the torsion angle makes from cis (C) ($\omega = 0°$) to $trans$ (T) ($\omega = 180°$). This allows for the definition of new, convenient collective variables. For instance, we define Ω as the sum of the cosines of the ω angles, which for an n-mer polyproline peptide with $n - 1$ prolyl bonds is:

$$\Omega_{n-mer} = \sum_{i=1}^{n-1} \cos \omega_i. \tag{2}$$

For a C (T) prolyl bond, $\cos \omega_i$ is $+1$ (-1) and therefore Ω_{n-mer} can take any of the following values: $-n + 1$, $-n + 3$, . . ., $n - 3$, or $n - 1$. This collective variable Ω gives the net balance of C and T prolyl bonds and obviously has some degeneracy. For a sequence with $n_b = n - 1$ bonds where each bond can be in either C or T, the number of conformations with n_C C bonds and n_T T bonds (with $n_b = n_C + n_T$) is $n_b!/(n_C!n_T!)$. Naturally, perfect PPI is characterized by $\Omega_{n-mer} = n - 1$ and perfect PPII by $\Omega_{n-mer} = -(n - 1)$.

Alternatively, one can consider the "interface" between bonds, and define a collective variable Λ as:

$$\Lambda_{n-mer} = \sum_{i=1}^{n-2} \cos(\omega_i + \omega_{i+1}). \tag{3}$$

For an n-mer, there are $n - 1$ prolyl bonds and $n - 2$ interfaces. If two neighboring bonds have the same dihedral angle ω then their interface is $\cos(\omega_i + \omega_{i+1}) = +1$, otherwise it is -1. Correspondingly, Λ_{n-mer} can take on any of the values $-n + 2$, $-n + 4$, . . ., $n - 4$, $n - 2$. Λ_{n-mer} removes some of the degeneracy associated with Ω. For $|\Omega| = n - 1$, there is only one value of Λ ($\Lambda = n - 2$); for $\Omega = 0$ (that exists only for odd values of n) there are ($n - 2$) values of Λ ; for $|\Omega| = m$ (with $m \neq n - 1$ and $m \neq 0$), there are $n - 1 - m$ values of Λ. Thus a typical free energy landscape in the (Ω, Λ) plane has a triangular shape.

Having the binary nature of dihedral angle ω, one can define many different ω-based collective variables such as Ω and Λ to identify different cis/trans patterns [6]. We note that all these dihedral angle ω-based collective variables can be generalized to any proline-containing peptide. Particularly, $\Omega = \sum_b \cos\omega_b$ (here sum runs over all the prolyl bonds) is a practical collective variable to "capture" different patterns of the cis/trans conformations in any proline-containing peptide. Particularly in the proline-rich peptides, Ω describes the slowest mode of the system.

2.2. Quantifying the PPII Propensity

To examine the concept of "intrinsic" PPII propensity of amino acids, one needs to (i) quantify the PPII content of amino acids in a system and (ii) distinguish between the intrinsic and non-intrinsic portion of this content. The latter requires an appropriate correlation analysis and the former requires not only a clear definition for the PPII secondary structure but also a practical statistical technique to measure the PPII content from a large conformational ensemble.

2.2.1. Identifying Secondary Structures

We used the (ϕ, ψ) dihedral angles to identify different regions [100] of the Ramachandran map [101]. According to this scheme, the α region is divided into two parts: α_R defined by $-120° < \psi < 90°$ and $-160° < \phi < -20°$ and α_L defined by $-50° < \psi < 110°$ and $20° < \phi < 160°$. The F region includes $-110° < \phi < -20°$ and ($90° < \psi < 180°$ or $-180° < \psi < -120°$). The β region consists of two parts: ($-180° < \phi < -110°$, $90° < \psi < 180°$ or $-180° < \psi < -120°$) and ($160° < \phi < 180°$ and $120° < \psi < 180°$) regions.

Although this delineates clear regions for the dihedrals of most residues, it turns out that there is considerable overlap between the populations of the F and β regions. In some cases the α_R region may overlap with both the F and β regions as well. In order to handle this situation, we used a clustering technique to identify the region of the conformations, rather than strictly enforcing the sharp boundaries of a given region[102, 103]. These two methods give identical answers for most dihedrals. However, at the borders, the clustering technique is deemed to be more accurate.

For non-proline amino acids, the PPII content is simply given by its F population, because the peptide bonds are all T. However, for proline both the C and T isomers fall in the F region. Since the C isomer is a signature of the PPI structure, these were not counted here since we were interested in the PPII content of the peptide *only*. Since an ideal PPII proline residue is in a trans conformation and also in the F region, one can find the probability of each residue being in the PPII conformation as $P(\text{PPII}) = P(\text{T}) \times P(\text{F}|\text{T})$. Similarly, the same holds true for a residue in the PPI configuration so that $P(\text{PPI}) = P(\text{C}) \times P(\text{F}|\text{C})$. Of course, then:

$$P(\text{F}) = P(\text{T}) \times P(\text{F}|\text{T}) + P(\text{C}) \times P(\text{F}|\text{C}) = P(\text{PPII}) + P(\text{PPI}). \quad (4)$$

This average $P(\text{F})$ can be used to estimate the PPII helical content of different polypeptides[55, 19, 56], not necessarily based on proline. In this context, the PPII helix refers only to the secondary structure of the polypeptides as identified by the values of ϕ and ψ torsion angles. As a matter of fact, although PPI proline residues are in cis conformation, they occupy the same region of Ramachandran plot as trans PPII prolines (on average $(-75°, 160°)$ and $(-75°, 146°)$ for PPI and PPII, respectively) and is considered as PPII content in this context.

2.2.2. Correlation Analysis

To quantify the changes in the conformational preferences of the peptides implied by different guest amino-acids we made use of the Odds Ratio[104] (OR) construction. The OR is a descriptive statistic that measures the strength of association, or non-independence, between two binary values. The OR is defined for two binary random variables (denoted as X and Y) as:

$$\text{OR} = \frac{p_{11}p_{00}}{p_{10}p_{01}}, \quad (5)$$

where $p_{ab} = p(X = a, Y = b)$ is the probability of the $(X = a, Y = b)$ event (with a and b taking on binary values of 0 and 1). For the purposes of this work, we can think of X and Y as being some characteristic properties describing the conformations of different residues. For example, the variables could be assigned values of 1 or 0 depending on whether the backbone dihedral angles of corresponding residue falls into a certain region of Ramachandran plot or not.

The usefulness of the OR in quantifying the influence of one binary random variable upon another can be readily seen. If the two variables are statistically independent, then $p_{ab} = p_a p_b$ so that $\text{OR} = 1$. In the opposite extreme case of $X = Y$ (complete dependence) both p_{10} and p_{01} are zero, and the OR is infinite. Similarly, for $X = \overline{Y}$ $p_{00} = p_{11} = 0$ rendering the OR zero. To summarize, an OR of unity indicates that the values of X are equally likely for both values of Y (*i.e.*, Y=1,0); an OR greater than unity indicates that the $X = 1$ is more likely when $Y = 1$, while an OR less than unity indicates that $X = 1$ is more likely when $Y = 0$.

It is convenient to recast the log of the OR in terms of free energy language. If one expresses the probability of the $(X = x, Y = y)$ events in terms of a free energy G_{xy}:

$$p_{xy} \propto \mathrm{e}^{-G_{xy}/k_B T}, \tag{6}$$

then the ratio of probabilities p_{xy}/p_{xz} translates into a free energy difference:

$$\ln \frac{p_{xy}}{p_{xz}} = -\,(G_{xy} - G_{xz})/\,k_B T. \tag{7}$$

Clearly, the logarithm of the OR then maps onto the difference of those differences, *i.e.*,

$$\Delta\Delta G = k_B T \ln \mathrm{OR}. \tag{8}$$

For the case of statistically independent properties, $\Delta\Delta G = 0$; otherwise, this quantity takes on either positive or negative values, whose magnitude depends on the mutual dependence between the two variables. The standard error of $\Delta\Delta G$ in its asymptotic approximation is:

$$SE(\Delta\Delta G) = k_B T \sqrt{\frac{1}{n_{11}} + \frac{1}{n_{00}} + \frac{1}{n_{10}} + \frac{1}{n_{01}}}. \tag{9}$$

in which n_{xy} is the total number of independent $(X = x, Y = y)$ events sampled.

While this development may be perceived as purely formal, the use of an OR analysis couched in terms of free energy language provides for a useful and intuitive measure of the inter-residual correlations such as host-guest correlations. In this context, OR-based correlation analysis is preferred over the more conventional linear correlation analysis partly because it eliminates the nonlinear noise associated with the fluctuation of dihedral angles. This noise may dominate the linear correlation results such that even substantial correlations may be completely ignored. The OR-based correlation analysis, combined with the clustering technique explained above takes into account both nonlinearity and multivariate components of amino acid correlations in a peptide chain.

2.3. Simulation Details

All the ABMD, HT-REMD and SMD simulations were carried both *in vacuo* and in implicit water[105, 106, 107]. We note that while simulations based on explicit waters are more desirable, they are (for the most part) precluded here because of their large computational costs. As a check, we were able to carry out selected SMD runs with explicit waters. The agreement between these runs and the corresponding implicit ones is very good [6]. Initial configurations consisted of the unfolded peptide, which was generated using the LEAP program of the AMBER v.9 simulation package. The simulations used the 1999 version of the Cornell *et al* force field[108]. We note that a recent study of several Amber force fields showed that both ff99 and ff99SB give very similar results for proline, with equilibrium structures that are consistent with experimental results[7, 109]. With regards to the impact of force field torsion parameters on proline simulations, studies[7, 109] suggest that changing these is unlikely to strongly impact the free energies and the distribution of the conformers. The most likely impact would be to change the free energy barriers between the different states. The leap-frog algorithm with a 1 fs timestep was used along with the Berendsen thermostat. For the *in vacuo* and implicit water calculations, there was no cutoff for the nonbonded interactions.

3. Polyproline Peptides

Polyproline peptides are characterized by a large number of stable conformers based on the cis/trans isomerization of the ω torsion angles. Here we review the structural and free energy characteristics of short polyproline peptides, *i.e.*, $Ace - (Pro)_n - Nme$, with n=2,..13, and examine the transition mechanisms between the PPI and PPII structures.

3.1. Free Energies of Polyproline Conformers

Figures 2-4 show typical examples of two-dimensional free energy maps as obtained from our ABMD simulations for a polyproline hexamer, nanomer, and tridecamer both *in vacuo* and in an implicit water environment. The figures plot the free energies in the (H, d_{end}), (Ω, R_g) and (Ω, Λ) phase space, respectively. These free energy maps show that the peptides are all characterized by stable conformational minima, whose number grows as the length of the peptide is increased. Qualitatively, the gas phase and implicit water results are similar, except that the implicit water shifts the equilibrium towards the PPII conformations.

Considering the free energy map shown in Fig. 2, one can classify the minima into three groups: (i) minima with relatively large end-to-end distance d_{end} and handedness $H < 0$ corresponding to left-handed polyproline helices; (ii) minima with relatively smaller d_{end} and $H > 0$ corresponding to right-handed polyproline helices; and (iii) minima centered around $H \approx 0$ which correspond to different compact structures. The effect of the solvent environment is particular evident for this particular free energy landscape. Considering the *in vacuo* results, for short hexamers the free energy favors the formation of PPII structures, as opposed to PPI. As the peptide length is increased, this trend reverses itself and PPI type structures are favored. The nanomer corresponds to an intermediate case, where the free energies of the PPI and PPII structures are approximately in balance. Such a change with peptide length has also been noted experimentally, particularly for polyproline in an alcohol environment. The free energy maps for polyproline peptides in *implicit water* is qualitatively similar, except that the left-handed PPII structure is favored over PPI structures for all chain lengths, in agreement with experimental results [30]. In such an implicit water environment, the free energy minima associated with PPII are of the same magnitude as those associated with the compact structures, and they form a "broad valley" in which the minima are separated by relatively low free energy barriers.

While the (d_{end}, H) results readily distinguish between PPI and PPII helices, they are not particularly useful for discriminating among different polyproline conformers because of the high degree of degeneracy associated with these collective variables. In other words, the numerical values of H and d_{end} of many isomers are too close together in order to allow for an unambiguous distinction. Hence, there are relatively 'few' minima on this free energy plot. More isomers are distinguishable on the (Ω, R_g) plots shown in Fig. 3. For an n-mer polypeptide, there are $n - 1$ prolyl bonds (ignoring the Ace-Pro bond), and so Ω runs between ± 5, ± 8 and ± 12 for the 6-mer, 9-mer, and 13-mer, respectively. The free energy minima associated with the Ω collective variable are elongated in the R_g direction, forming a set of narrow valleys. These are a reflection of the degeneracy of Ω and the underlying structures they represent. For example, the flipping of a single bond within an all-trans helix does not modify the helical structure if the bond is near one of the ends, but produces a sharp turn when it is near the peptide center. For the nanomer, the deepest minima correspond to globular and PPII structures. Since the PPII-like helices are more stretched, they have more flexibility in terms of R_g, unlike the PPI

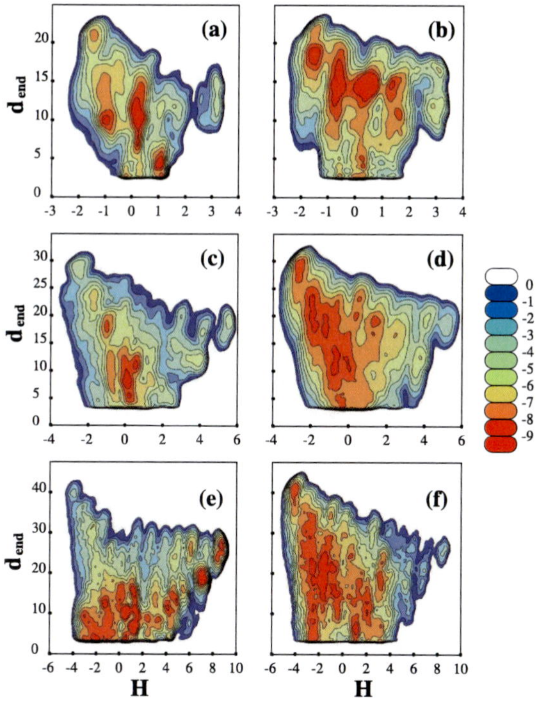

Figure 2. The (H, d_{end}) free energy landscapes in $kcal/mol$ for a polyproline (a,b) hexamer, (c,d) nanomer, and (e,f) tridecamer peptide *in vacuo* (a,c,e) and implicit water (b,d,f).

structures which are much more rigid. This translates into a net decrease of the elongation of as one moves from PPII to PPI. Also, while the general shape of the free energy plots are quite similar for the *in vacuo* and implicit water results, it is evident that the latter favors PPII-like structures.

Further distinction of the different isomers is evident on the (Ω, Λ) plots shown in Fig. 4. For a peptide of length n, there are $n - 1$ prolyl bonds, and $n - 2$ "interfaces" between them. For our 6-, 9-, and 13-mer peptides, Λ therefore varies between ± 4, ± 7, and ± 11, respectively. Here, the minima associated with the maximal numerical value of Λ is associated with either a PPI (positive Ω) or PPII (negative Ω) helix, since both of these structures have no cis/trans interface. By contrast, $\Omega = 0$ and Λ taking on its most negative value correspond to a situation where all the cis/trans bonds alternate. Overall, the

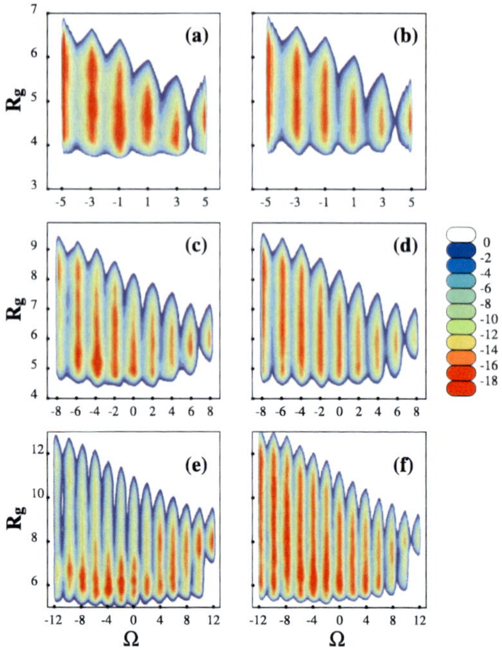

Figure 3. The (Ω, R_g) free energy landscapes in $kcal/mol$ for a polyproline (a,b) hexamer, (c,d) nanomer, and (e,f) tridecamer peptide *in vacuo* (a,c,e) and implicit water (b,d,f).

free energy minima on these maps are distributed in a triangular or wedge-like pattern.

Table I summarizes all the free energy minima for the polyproline dimer to tridecamer, as obtained from different collective variables. Both *in vacuo* and implicit solvent results are given. The free energy results as obtained from the different collective variables are in good agreement with each other: for the most part, numerical values differ from each other by less than 1 kcal/mol. In terms of general trends, for *in vacuo* peptides, the PPII structure in short peptides is favored over PPI. For short peptides, the free energy difference $f(\text{PPI}) - f(\text{PPII})$ increases from about 0.5 kcal/mol for a dimer up to about 7.5 kcal/mol for a tetramer and then it decreases with increasing lengths of chains. Computed values of the free energy difference based on the Ω map are 3.5 kcal/mol for the heptamer, 0.7 kcal/mol for the octamer, and 0.5 kcal/mol for the nanomer. For longer lengths, there appears to be a crossover and PPI structures are favored.

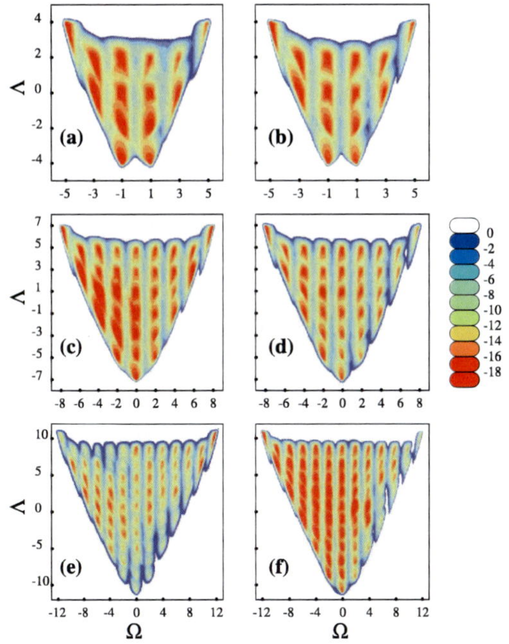

Figure 4. The (Ω, Λ) free energy landscapes in $kcal/mol$ for a polyproline (a,b) hexamer, (c,d) nanomer, and (e,f) tridecamer peptide *in vacuo* (a,c,e) and implicit water (b,d,f).

Thus, for a 13-mer, the free energy difference favors PPI and is estimated to be about 6.4 kcal/mol[5]. For short peptides up to a tetramer, the PPII structure is also the global minimum. For longer peptides, the global minimum is associated with a "melted", globular like peptide structure. However, the difference between the PPI minimum and the global disordered minimum also decreases with polymer chain length (for the 9-mer this difference is 5.69 kcal/mol while for the 13-mer, it is 1.38 kcal/mol). Thus, it is quite likely that PPI becomes the global minimum as the peptide length is increased even further.

The free energy maps were also computed in implicit water. In this case, the PPII structure is always associated with the global minimum and $f(\text{PPI}) - f(\text{PPII})$ increases with polymer chain. What is the origin of the different behavior in gas phase and in water? The structure of polyproline is such that the nitrogen atom of the prolyl bond is precluded from engaging in hydrogen bonding. This not only determines the structure of the helices, but also

Table 1. Free energy difference between PPI and PPII structures [f(PPI)-f(PPII)] in $kcal/mol$ as obtained from different ABMD maps

	Δf $(kcal/mol)$ *in vacuo*			Δf $(kcal/mol)$ in implicit water		
n	Ω	(Ω, d_{end})	(Ω, Λ)	Ω	(Ω, d_{end})	(Ω, Λ)
2	0.55	0.50	-	1.90	1.33	-
3	4.31	3.85	4.29	3.38	3.06	3.20
4	7.07	7.47	7.58	4.20	4.44	4.89
5	5.84	6.33	5.96	4.02	5.30	4.11
6	5.26	5.31	5.98	4.86	5.82	5.31
7	3.49	-	-	6.12	-	-
8	0.69	-	-		6.05 -	-
9	0.49	1.92	1.24	6.57	6.47	6.08
13	-	-6.02	-6.65	-	7.97	8.05

the interaction with solvents. The cis/trans conformations that characterize the two helices have an effect on the orientation of the carboxyl groups $C = O$: in PPI these groups are almost parallel to the axis of the compact helix and are shielded from the solvent by proline rings; in PPII the $C = O$ groups are mainly perpendicular to the axis of the helix, and since the helix is more elongated, the carboxyl oxygen atom is more exposed to solvents. One can expect, therefore, that the more this entity interacts with a solvent, the more PPII will be favored over PPI. In water, this interaction is such that PPII is always favored, which is in contrast to the gas phase where there is no interaction at all. This is also consistent with the behavior of polyproline peptides in other solvent environments. We have simulated a nanomer in explicit hexane and 1-propanol as an example of interactions with a nonpolar solvent and yet another polar solvent[5]. Results indicate that PPII is favored in the hexane environment, and PPI in the alcohol environment, with a free energy difference (f(PPI) $-$ f(PPII)) – based on averaging three independent sets of collective variables – of 19.3 and -7.1 kcal/mol, respectively. These results are in agreement with experimental conclusions based on the CD spectra of proline oligopeptides[30] which show the stability of the PPI helix is enhanced in aliphatic alcohols with longer chains.

Table II presents the five most probable conformations and their percentages as obtained from HT-REMD equilibrium sampling in implicit water. In

Table 2. The five most probable structures for hexamer, heptamer, octomer, and nanomer polyproline peptides in implicit water along with their occurrence percentage (bracketed), as estimated by the HT-REMD method

Hexamer	Heptamer	Octamer	Nanomer
TTTTT (45 %)	TTTTTT (35 %)	TTTTTTT (28 %)	TTTTTTTT (22 %)
TTCTT (11 %)	TTCTTT (12 %)	TTTCTTT (8 %)	TTTCTTTT (6 %)
TTTTC (9 %)	TTTCTT (7 %)	TTCTTTT (6 %)	TTTTTCTT (6 %)
TCTTT (7 %)	TTTTTC (5 %)	TTTTCTT (6 %)	TTTTCTTT (5 %)
CTTTT (6 %)	TCTTTT (4 %)	TTTTTTC (5 %)	TTCCTTTT (5 %)

principle, the population distributions of the conformers may be obtained from their relative free energies. In practice, this may not be the most convenient way of obtaining these quantities, since this requires an exponentiation of the free energy differences which magnifies the errors inherent in these quantities tremendously. Hence, we make use of HT-REMD simulations as a powerful, complementary alternative. In implicit water both ABMD and HT-REMD results confirm PPII as the most probable structure. The second most probable structure is always PPII with only a single peptide bond in the cis conformation that typically is found in the center. We also note that while PPII is always the most probably structure in implicit water, its percentage decreases with increasing chain length: *i.e.,* 93 %, 84 %, 75 %, 63 %, 45 %, 35 %, 28 % and 22 % for a dimer through nanomer, respectively (not all the data shown in Table II).

3.2. Transition Mechanisms

To examine the transition mechanisms between PPI and PPII, SMD simulations were used with the successive flipping of the ω dihedral angles. Since it is not possible to exhaustively examine all possible transition pathways and mechanisms, we concentrated on the most likely mechanisms which were identified as the ones that contribute the most to the sum in ΔF in the Jarzynski relation. These correspond to pathways that require the least amount of work. Specifically, we focused on different zipper-like mechanisms, for which changes take place via the successive switching of neighboring prolyl bonds. These include: a zipper-like mechanism starting from the forward, N-terminal for the PPII→PPI transition (and the opposite for the PPI→PPII transition) which we label zipper(N), such that the intermediate conformation in either direction would take the form Ace−CCC...TTT−Nme; a zipper-like mechanism starting from the reverse, C-terminal for the PPII→PPI transition and the opposite for the PPI→PPII transition which we label zipper(C), such that the intermediate conformation would take the form Ace−TTT...CCC−Nme); a zipper-like mechanism starting from the center and moving outwards for the PPII→PPI transition and opposite for the reverse transition which we label in-out, such that the intermediate conformation would take the form Ace−TT...CCC...TT−Nme; a zipper-like mechanism starting from both ends, and working its way inward for the PPII→PPI transition, and opposite for the reverse transition which we label out-in, such that the intermediate conformation would take the form Ace−CC...TTT...CC−Nme. Additionally, we considered mechanisms that involve changing the prolyl bonds at random, and an "en-masse" mechanism where all the bonds are changed simultaneously.

Clearly, there is some ambiguity in how the in-out and out-in mechanisms can be implemented. For example, one can flip either two bonds at a time *simultaneously*, or only one at a time. For the latter, the order of bond flipping provides for a further degree of freedom. In most cases, the alternative flipping of bonds in either direction required the least amount of work, and was therefore used for the out-in and in-out mechanisms.

Figure 5 shows typical work profiles obtained from SMD simulations for a polyproline nanomer *in vacuo*. One can see a trend in which in-out and zipper(C) mechanisms are associated with the least amount of work. Similar results were also obtained for other polyproline systems both *in vacuo* and implicit/explicit water[6].

While these zipper-based mechanisms appear to be the most likely, an important question remains as to where the initial bond rotation takes place. In these PPII→PPI transition simulations, the amidated end and/or middle bonds appear to be good options. Although the difference between the required work by zipper(C) and zipper(N) is more significant in gas phase, it is still recognizable in implicit water. This is consistent with the results from enzymatic hydrolysis kinetics experiments on polyproline in aqueous solution [110, 111] but opposite to the results from the NMR experiments on polyproline in D_2O solution[112] and a theoretical conclusion based on *ab initio* free energy calculations[74].

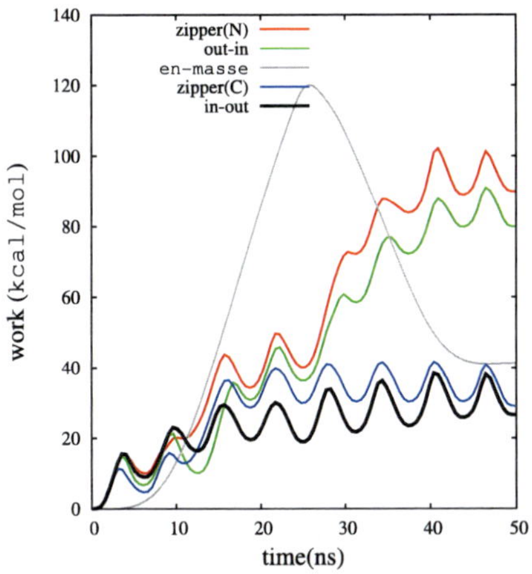

Figure 5. The work (W) (required for a typical PPII→PPI transition) versus time for a nanomer in *in vacuo*. Different mechanisms are characterized by different colors.

4. PPII Propensity of Non-proline Amino Acids

There has been considerable debate about the intrinsic PPII propensity of amino acid residues in denatured polypeptides. Experimentally, this scale is based on the behavior of guest amino acid residues placed in the middle of proline-based hosts[54, 55, 56, 57, 58, 59, 60]. We recently examined this issue with classical MD combined with REMD, which allows for a comprehensive analysis of the conformational equilibria of the proline hosts with a single and multiple amino acid guests [8, 9]. The tracked structural characteristics include the secondary structural motifs of the peptides based on the Ramachandran plots, and the cis/trans isomerization of the prolyl bonds. We find that these peptides share similar structural features, and that a population analysis of secondary structure motifs (residue by residue) shows that the guest residues (other than Pro) do not favor the F region. We find that there is no need to invoke an "intrinsic PPII propensity" in order to explain the experimental results. Rather, these may be understood in terms of the following. (i) As it is well-known[66, 113], proline peptides are conformationally restricted by their pyrrolidine rings, and by steric interactions with neighbouring prolines. In fact, a proline restricts the dihedrals of a preceding residue to $50^\circ < \psi < 180^\circ$ (except for Gly), forcing the preceding residue to be in either a β or F region, according to the value of ϕ. In the present host-guest setup, there is a statistical, Boltzmann-weighted distribution of conformations, with the highest percentage of the guest population found in the β region; (ii) The cis/trans proline ratio depends on the sequence surrounding the proline residue[66]. For this particular set of host-guest peptides, we find that every guest (Pro, Tyr, and Trp excepted) increases the trans content of the prolyl bonds. The guest amino acids therefore are not characterized by any PPII propensity, but rather collaborate with their own *intrinsic trans* propensity, to destabilize the cis isomers of the proline hosts, which results in a *de facto* net PPII increase; (iii) there is a local correlation between the dihedral angles of the guest and the proline residue immediately preceding the guest. We find that the degree to which the guest influences this proline (and visa versa) is conveniently described in terms of an odds ratio analysis.

Simulations were carried out for the following peptides: Ace$-$(Pro)$_3-$X$_n-$(Pro)$_3-$Gly$-$Tyr$-$NH$_2$ (denoted as PX$_n$P or PXP for $n = 1$), with the guests X_n taken from the following list of amino acids: P(Pro), Q(Gln), D(Asp), A(Ala), R(Arg), E(Glu), K(Lys), G(Gly), L(Leu), F(Phe), S(Ser), M(Met), C(Cys), H(His), N(Asn), T(Thr), I(Ile), V(Val), W(Trp), and Y(Tyr). Here, n ranges from 1 to 7 for X=A,Q, (1 to 3) X=V,N, and only 1 for the rest of amino acids. In each case, we refer to the first three proline residues as P^1, P^2, and P^3, and to the last three as P^4, P^5, and P^6, respectively. The guest residues are then labeled as Ace$-$P$^1-$P$^2-$P$^3-$X$_n^1-$X$_n^2$ $-$ $\cdots-$X$_n^n-$P$^4-$P$^5-$P$^6-$Gly$-$Tyr-NH$_2$. For PXP peptides, X simply refers to the only guest amino acid. We note that the choice of PX_nP peptides investigated is motivated by the experiments[55, 56, 57, 58, 59, 60].

As already mentioned, applicability of regular MD to this system is limited because of the slow cis/trans isomerization of the prolyl bonds. These transitions correspond to the changes of the ω torsion angles between $\omega = 0°$ (C) and $\omega = 180°$ (T). We thus "capture" the different patterns of the cis/trans conformations with the Ω collective variable. Here the ACE-Pro bond is also included, therefore Ω ranges from $-n$ (all-trans) to n (all-cis) for a proline-based peptide involving n proline residues. We performed 100 ns of HT-REMD simulations in implicit water with 24 replicas of each peptide for enhanced equilibrium sampling (for the details, see previous Section). We used the one-dimensional biasing potentials generated by ABMD method for the polyprolines with the same number of prolyl bonds included in the definition of Ω. We note that we performed short ABMD simulations to refine the biasing potentials for the specific systems, prior to the "production" runs in which coordinates of the unbiased $T = 300$ K replica were sampled every picosecond for the statistical analysis.

4.1. PPII Content

Having collected 10^5 equilibrium samples for each PX_nP peptide with the HT-REMD simulations, we have analyzed their structural properties with a focus on the PPII content. The results are summarized in Tables III and IV and Figures 6 and 7. Ramachandran plots for selected residues are shown in Figure 6. Specifically, the figure presents Ramachandran maps of (a) P^1, (b) X(=P), and (c) P^6 prolines in PPP and X in (d) PQP, (e) PAP, and (f) PVP, X^3 in (g) PQ_3P, (h) PA_3P, and (i) PV_3P. Each pixel represents a $1° \times 1°$ bin, whose intensity represents its relative population, ranging from 1,2,. . . ,9, and 10 or more conformations, sampled in our simulations. Blue, yellow, grey, and pink clusters identify the F, β, α_R, and α_L regions.

Table III quantifies the F and PPII content of each residue for select PX_nP peptides. Since steric interactions constrain the structure of neighboring prolines, all the proline residues which are followed by another proline, *i.e.*, P^1, P^2, P^4, P^5 (and P^3 in PP_1P), are restricted to the F region of their Ramachandran plots. A typical illustration of this is given in Fig.6a,b, which shows results for residue (a) P^1 and (b) guest X=P of PPP, About 94-100 % of these residues fall into the F region on the Ramachandran plots, but these numbers drop by 15 to 25 % when the PPII content is considered (*i.e.*, when the cis isomers are excluded). P^6 differs from the other residues since it is not followed by another proline. Its dihedrals are distributed between the F and α_R regions (Fig. 6c). Table III also gives the variation of the PPII (F) contents of P^6, which ranges between 33 (35) to 49 (53) %, depending on the guests. When P^3 is followed by a guest X≠P, its F and PPII content decreases dramatically. Table III also gives PPII content of the terminal glycine and tyrosine. Since glycine is quite flexible, it explores more regions of the Ramachandran plot, with now only 6-9 % in the F-region. For tyrosine, all four regions are available, and about 32 to 38 % of these residues fall in the F region. There appears to be little variation of these numbers with respect to the type of guest, presumably because of the relatively large distance of the peptide tail to its center.

Table 3. PPII content and F content (bracketed) of different residues (as a percentage), along with their averages for select PX_nP peptides

peptide	P^1,P^2,P^4,P^5	P^3	P^6	G	Y	average X_n^i	$X_n^1,X_n^2,...,X_n^n$	**average**
PA_1P	81 (99)	14 (18)	37 (40)	6	37	27	27	**50 (58)**
PA_3P	83 (98)	7 (7)	37 (41)	7	33	21	4,10,49	**43 (49)**
PA_7P	88 (98)	10 (10)	41 (44)	6	36	16	4,8,19,11,18,12,42	**37 (40)**
PQ_1P	81 (98)	16 (22)	33 (35)	6	38	27	27	**50 (58)**
PQ_3P	83 (98)	3 (4)	37 (40)	7	35	21	2,6,57	**44 (49)**
PQ_7P	89 (98)	8 (9)	46 (48)	7	35	11	2,1,12,3,5,10,44	**35 (38)**
PV_1P	80 (99)	13 (17)	34 (37)	7	36	22	22	**48 (57)**
PV_3P	81 (98)	7 (11)	38 (43)	7	33	17	3,12,35	**42 (49)**
PN_1P	78 (100)	18 (22)	42 (44)	6	38	11	11	**47 (58)**
PN_3P	80 (99)	5 (6)	48 (50)	7	37	12	5,17,15	**41 (48)**
PP_1P	74 (99)	70 (100)	41 (46)	6	32	51 (99)	51 (99)	**55 (76)**

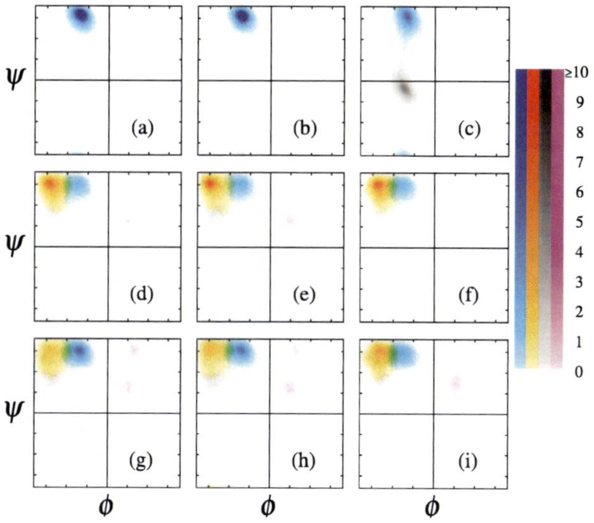

Figure 6. Ramachandran maps of (a) N-terminal, (b) middle, and (c) C-terminal prolines in PPP along with the Ramachandran maps of the guest amino acids (preceding a proline) in (d) PQP, (e) PAP, (f) PVP, (g) PQ_3P, (h) PA_3P, and (i) PV_3P. Each pixel represents a $1^\circ \times 1^\circ$ bin, whose intensity represents its relative population, ranging from 1,2,. . .,9, and 10 or more conformations, sampled in our simulations. Blue, yellow, grey, and pink clusters identify F, β, α_R, and α_L regions.

Ramachandran plots of the select guest residues are shown in Figs 6b,d-i for PX_nP peptides. For the C-terminal guest – which is immediately followed by P^4 – only a very small population falls outside the F-β regions, which effectively merge together. In contrast, the further the guest is from P^4, the less PPII content it has (not shown in the Figure). In particular, the guest immediately following P^3 typically has the lowest PPII content. Table III gives a quantitative measure of the F content of the guest residues. For the X_n^n residues, the PPII content can be as high as 57 % (Q_3^3) or as low as 11 % (N_1^1). For the X_n^i, $i < n$, the PPII content is always less than 20 %, even less than 10 % in most cases when alanine is excluded. In all cases the X_n^n residue has the highest PPII content, simply because of the steric restrictions imposed on its ψ dihedral angle. Comparing results for alanine and glutamine, we see that the remaining residues are all characterized by a smaller PPII content. In the case of glutamine, this "fall-off" is relatively steep.

Clearly, the PPII content drops as the number of guest amino acids is increased. The fall-off is most substantial for the PQ_nP peptides. These features are in agreement with the CD experimental results[57, 58, 60]. In the case of alanine with $n < 4$, this decrease is offset by an increase in the PPII content of the alanine residue preceding P^4, which actually increases, *i.e.*, 27 %, 39 % and 49 % for PA_1P, PA_2P, and PA_3P respectively. Numerically, these two effects roughly balance each other for the alanine guest peptides, and so there is only a modest decrease in the average PPII content of the guests with increasing guest number, *i.e.*, 3 % decrease for each additional guest. This is in agreement with the experimental conclusion that PA_1P, PA_2P, and PA_3P have very similar CD spectra[57]. However, the simulations show that this is not due to the intrinsic PPII propensity of alanine itself. Although the average PPII content of guests does not decrease dramatically, only the C-terminal guest that is under steric restrictions has a considerable PPII content. For A_n, $n > 3$, the PPII content of this guest does not change much and the decrease in the average PPII content of the guests remains modest when the whole peptide is considered. However, this decrease cannot be ignored because now at least half the peptide consists of non-proline amino acids which have no real PPII content. This is consistent with the CD spectra of multiple-alanine guest peptides[58], which also examined peptides with up to seven guests.

In terms of the cis/trans isomerization, our results show that there is an increase in the T content of the prolyl bonds as guest amino acids are added. This increase in the T content of the prolyl bonds was also observed in single-amino acid guest peptides, and partially compensates for the decrease in PPII content with increasing guest number.

In summary, the examined host-guest peptides all share many structural characteristics which depend on their location within a given peptide. Hence, the Ramachandran plots of different amino acid guests appear to be quite similar, provided that they represent the same residue within the given multiple-guest peptide. In terms of the PPII content, the guests immediately preceding residue P^4 are constrained by the proline ring of P^4 to the F and β regions. These guests typically have the highest F (PPII) content. For a fixed guest number, the F-β content decreases while the α_R content increases as one moves from P^4 to P^3.

4.2. Host-Guest Correlations

Since P^3 and the guest residue X^1 show the most significant variation in terms of the F and PPII content, it is natural to explore the correlation between the two neighboring residues. This correlation is most conveniently expressed in terms of the odds ratio (OR) construction previously reviewed. We have carried out a full population analysis, and calculated the OR based on whether or not a given residue (here P^3 and X^1) is in either the PPII conformation, or not (*i.e.*, being both in the F region of the Ramachandran plots and having a trans isomer).

Based on the numerical values of PPII-based OR calculated for P^3 and X^1 residues, one can classify the guests as having strong, intermediate, or weak correlations by means of (arbitrary) introduced cutoffs. Using the PPII-based OR, we define guests as being strongly correlated if their $OR > 2$. Guests with intermediate correlations are those with $1 < OR \leq 2$; and weakly correlated guests are those with $0 < OR \leq 1$. Table IV summarizes the resulting grouping of guest amino acids (for all single-guest peptides) according to their nature. Typically, negatively charged amino acids, positively charged Lys, and the polar amino acids Gln and Ser make for highly correlated guests, while the rest of the polar amino acids and Arg are guests with intermediate correlations. Hydrophobic amino acids result in guests of intermediate or weak correlations, except for Gly and the small hydrophobic amino acid Ala, which show quite strong P_3-X correlations. For those amino acids whose OR falls near the cutoffs, the character of the correlation should only be taken as indicative, since their classification is obviously sensitive to the chosen cutoffs, which may be altered, for instance, in the presence of explicit waters. Finally, we note that an OR less than unity indicates a *de facto* anti-correlation, as observed for instance in Tyr.

A comparison between the experimental PPII content [56] of the PXP peptides against the corresponding $\Delta\Delta G$'s is shown in Fig.7. This plot clearly shows that there is a linear correlation between the experimental and simulation results, with a correlation coefficient of $R = 0.85$. This correlation – which is strictly based on th $P_3 - X$ OR – does not include any nonlocal cis/trans isomerization effects. When comparing the experimental and simulation data, it is sensible to say that our $\Delta\Delta G$ correlates with the maximum molar ellipticity (which is related to PPII content, but is not exactly proportional to it). Although the initial PX_nP experiments were interpreted in the context of a PPII propensity scale for each amino acid as determined by the relative heights of an intensity peak in the CD spectrum[55, 56], the more recent experimental

Table 4. Grouping of amino acids according to their nature and the strength of the P_3-X correlation. Note that histidine is assumed to be protonated

	charged				
OR	(-)	(+)	polar	hydrophobic	small
$OR > 2$	E D	K	Q S	-	A G
$1 < OR \leq 2$	-	R H	N T C	L F M W	-
$0 < OR \leq 1$	-	-	-	V Y I	-

studies[57, 58, 59, 60] focus more on a relative qualitative comparison.

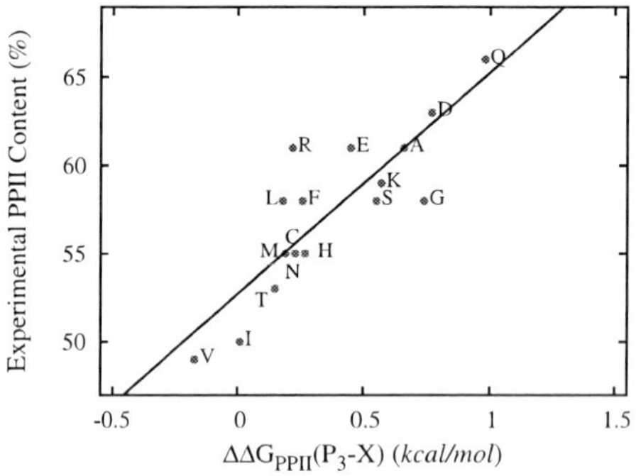

Figure 7. Experimental values[56] of the PPII content plotted against $\Delta\Delta G$, computed from the odds ratio of PPII for the P_3 and X residues in PXP peptides (X≠P,Y,W). Labels identify the guest amino acids. The correlation coefficient between the two data is $R = 0.85$. Note that histidine is assumed to be protonated.

While we are encouraged by the qualitative agreement with the experimental results, our interpretation of these results is rather different. First, we consider how the experimental notion of an *intrinsic* PPII propensity in the case of Ala comes about[55]. Since the CD spectra only reflect statistical ensemble *averages*, it is not possible to uniquely infer the properties of individual residues from these averages, unless some assumptions are made. In brief, it is assumed that: (i) From the CD measurements for PPII content, it is estimated that a well-behaved PPII residue will contribute about 11% to the overall PPII content. Thus, a lower bound of the PPII content will be 44%, attributed to the contributions of $P_{1,2,4,5}$; (ii) Since the proline closest to the C-terminal (*i.e.*, residue P_6) is not restricted by a following proline, it is assumed that this residue is free to adopt any conformation available to proline. Thus, the expectation is that P_6 does not contribute much to the overall PPII content; (iii) The C-terminal Tyr is not expected to contain any significant PPII content, while the case of the C-terminal Gly is unclear; (iv) Alanine is not expected to have much effect on its preceding proline. Thus, the P_3 residue is expected to adopt all conformations generally accessible to proline, unless long-range interactions (which extend beyond the nearest neighbor residues) favor a PPII helical conformation. The latter is not considered as a possibility; (v) Since the experimentally measured PPII content is 61% for PAP, of which 44% is accounted for by P_1, P_2, P_4, and P_5, and since all the other residues are not expected to make any significant contribution to the PPII content, "one is left to conclude that an isolated alanine has a high propensity to adopt this conformation" [55].

By contrast, simulations can produce extensive and accurate statistical data on *each* residue, and therefore serve to highlight the pitfalls of inferring individual system properties from a statistical ensemble average. Consider the F (PPII) content of PAP at 27° C, which was found to be 57% (48%), respectively. How do our observations differ from those of the experiments: (i) Indeed, residues P_1, P_2, P_4, and P_5 all make similar contributions. These are 11% (9%) per residue, and therefore account for 77% (63%) of the total F (PPII) content of the PAP peptide at 27° C; (ii) Residue P_6 contributes 4.4% (4%); or 7.8% (8.3%) of the total peptide F (PPII) content; (iii) The C-terminal Tyr also has a considerable PPII content: 4% for the residue, which represents 8.3% of total peptide PPII content. However, the C-terminal Gly has a negligible PPII content: 0.5% for the residue, which represents 1% of total peptide PPII content; (iv) Residue P_3 contributes 2% (1.4%), which represents 3.5% (2.9%) of the total peptide F (PPII) content; (v) Finally, the Ala residue contributes only 2.3%, or 4.8% to the total peptide PPII content. In other words, when each residue is considered individually, then the contribution of the Ala guest to the overall PPII content of the peptide is seen to be relatively modest, in agreement with the previous calculations of Vila *et al.* [19]. Indeed, as already noted, for PAP only 21% of the guest Ala is to be found in the F region, while 77% is found in the β region.

So, rather than invoking an intrinsic PPII propensity for the guest residues,

we argue that the behavior of amino acids in a proline host environment may be explained in terms of the following two properties which so far have not been considered:
(i) a local correlation between the dihedral angles of residues P_3 and X, which may be described in terms of an OR;
(ii) a non-local correlation between the cis/trans conformers of the peptide bonds.

Turning to proline-based peptides with multiple guests, we too find here that our computational results are in good qualitative agreement with the CD-based experiments[55, 56, 57, 58, 59, 60]. Experimentally, peptides with 2, 3, 5, and 7 guest alanines have been investigated[55, 56, 57, 58, 59]. The studies concluded that multiple-guest alanines also possess a high PPII content, and that a short sequence of alanine can adopt the PPII conformation[57]. The high PPII propensity of alanine is attributed to its small side chain[57] that does not interfere with solvation since it is believed that backbone solvation favors PPII conformation[36]. In contrast, bulky β-branched amino acids such as valine prevent optimal solvation by partially burying the backbone and therefore do not favor PPII[57].

Multiple glutamine guests have been also studied[57, 60] often by comparing these peptides to PP_1P and PN_nP peptides since N(Asn) is an amino acid similar to glutamine that does not favor the formation of a PPII helix. Amongst the different non-proline guests, glutamine has the highest PPII propensity of the proline-based systems with a single host. As the number of glutamines increases, the PPII content decreases dramatically when compared to alanine[57]. Nevertheless, the PPII content of glutamine tracts consisting of up to 15 residues remains significant, such that the 223-228 nm maximum CD spectral peak of a $PQ_{15}P$ is higher than that of PN_3P[60]. However, as the number of glutamine residues is increased, the intensity of the positive band decreases, indicating that the propensity to form PPII structure is local for glutamine[60]. The high PPII propensity of glutamine is hypothesized to be related to the high conformational entropy of its side chain and/or a hydrogen bond between the glutamine side chain and the backbone carbonyl oxygen[60]. Asparagine, in other hand, is too short to form this supposed hydrogen bond. We note that examining our structures, we did not find any evidence for this hydrogen bond in our glutamine-containing proline-based peptides. Chellgren *et al.* [60] concluded that glutamine residues in monomeric polyglutamine have a significant propensity to adopt PPII, although not necessarily in long continuous helical stretches.

Instead, they proposed a model in which monomeric polyglutamine chains exist as a dynamic ensemble of conformations consisting of short stretches of PPII helical structure interspersed with other structures.

5. Conclusion

In this chapter, we reviewed a number of simulation studies dealing primarily with the structure and free energies of pure polyproline peptides, and polyproline peptides with amino acid guests. These investigations shed light not only on proline systems, but may also be viewed as a paradigm for molecules whose conformational space contains both left- and right-handed helices. To this end, the simulations were based on MD with the ABMD method for calculating free energy landscapes complemented with HT-REMD and SMD simulations.

In terms of the pure polyproline peptides, the free energy landscapes of short peptides both *in vacuo* and in implicit waters were investigated, along with nanomers in explicit hexane and 1-propanol. The free energies were all calculated as a function of several relevant collective variables: handedness, radius of gyration, end-to-end distance, and the variables Ω, Λ and Γ associated specifically with the cis/trans isomerization of the peptide bond. We presented a sequence and residue based analysis of the polyproline conformations (for $n = 2, \ldots, 9$) based on a large number of equilibrium conformations sampled by HT-REMD method. We also considered pathways of minimum free energy through these landscapes, along which transitions between PPI and PPII forced via SMD.

General trends are as follows. *In vacuo*, the stability of cis PPI is enhanced with an increased peptide length; in implicit water, the trans PPII is always favored. This means that cooperativity or inter-residue interaction is more favorable in PPI than PPII. Pure PPI and PPII are just one of the minima in the phase space, with many other minima corresponding to other stable subpopulations whose representative structures are characterized in terms of the cis/trans bonds. These results are in good agreement with experimental observations. Our results complement the PET experimental results of Doose *et al*, with regards to the existence of stable heterogeneous subpopulation of polyproline conformers [16]. More importantly, by providing detailed free energy landscapes in terms of different collective variables, we are able to characterize the distribution of different isomers, along with probable transition paths and accompanying free energies.

In terms of transition mechanisms, these are associated with different pathways in phase space, some extreme examples being the case when all bonds rotate together, a melting and re-ordering mechanism, and a set of more probable zipper-like mechanisms. Based on a consideration of the work performed, zipper-like mechanisms starting from either the center of the peptide or the amidated end appear to be the most likely mechanism in the PPII→PPI transition in the longer peptides.

We also investigated the structural characteristics of proline-based oligopeptides in a host-guest setting. Specifically, the equilibrium structures of PX_nP peptides, as obtained from HT-REMD simulations, were analyzed. The features probed include the cis/trans isomerization of the prolyl bonds, the puckering of the pyrrolidine rings of the proline residues, and the secondary structural motifs associated with the distribution of dihedral angles of the Ramachandran plots for each residue. The cis/trans isomerization of each peptide structure was explicitly tracked when calculating the PPII content. We do not find significant evidence of an intrinsic PPII propensity for the guest amino acids. The experimentally observed changes in the height of the maximum molar ellipticity at 228 nm of the CD spectra, assumed to be proportional to the PPII content, may be explained in terms of the following observations: (i) Steric interactions produced by the proline rings[66, 113] cause a given proline to restrict the preceding residue to $50 < \psi < 180$ (except for Gly), forcing the preceding residue to be in either a β or F region, according to the value of ϕ; (ii) The net increase in *prolyl* trans content introduced by guests (other than Pro, Tyr and Trp) in the host peptide precludes some of the PPP cis isomers and effectively results in a net ($trans$) PPII increase; (iii) There is a local correlation between the dihedral angles of the guest, and the proline residue immediately preceding the guest, which may be effectively quantified by means of an OR analysis.

References

[1] Adzhubei, A. A.; Sternberg, M. J. E. *J. Mol. Biol.* 1993, 229, 472-493.

[2] Pawson, T. *Nature* 1995, 373, 573-580.

[3] Cohen, G.; Ren, R.; Baltimore, D. *Cell* 1995, 80, 237-248.

[4] Adzhubei, A. A.; Sternberg, M. J. E. *Protein Science* 1994, 3, 2395-2410.

[5] Moradi, M.; Babin, V.; Roland, C.; Darden, T.; Sagui, C. *Proc. Natl. Aca. Sci. USA* 2009, 106, 20746.

[6] Moradi, M.; Babin, V.; Roland, C.; Sagui, C. *J. Chem. Phys.* 2010, 133, 125104.

[7] Moradi, M.; Lee, J.-G.; Babin, V.; Roland, C.; Sagui, C. *Int. J. Quantum Chem.* 2010, 110, 2865 – 2879.

[8] Moradi, M.; Babin, V.; Sagui, C.; Roland, C. *Biophysical J.* 2011, 100, 1083 – 1093.

[9] Moradi, M.; Babin, V.; Sagui, C.; Roland, C. *J. Phys. Chem. B* 2011, 115, 8645-8656.

[10] Stryer, L.; Haugland, R. P. *Proc. Natl. Acad. Sci. USA.* 1967, 58, 719-726.

[11] Jacob, J.; Baker, B.; Bryant, G. R.; Cafiso, D. S. *Biophys. J.* 1999, 77, 1086-1092.

[12] Watkins, L. P.; Chang, H.; Yang, H. *J. Phys. Chem. A* 2006, 110, 5191-5203.

[13] Sahoo, H.; Roccatano, D.; Hennig, A.; Nau, W. M. *J. Am. Chem. Soc.* 2007, 129, 9762-9772.

[14] Schuler, B.; Lipman, E. A.; Steinbach, P. J.; Kumke, M.; Eaton, W. A. *Proc. Nat. Acad. Sci. U. S.A.* 2005, 102, 9754-9759.

[15] Best, R. B.; Merchant, K. A.; Gopich, I. V.; Schuler, B.; Bax, A.; Eaton, W. A. *Proc. Nat. Acad. Sci. U. S.A.* 2007, 104, 18964-18969.

[16] Doose, S.; Neuweiler, H.; Barsch, H.; Sauer, M. *Proc. Natl. Acad. Sci. USA.* 2007, 104, 17400-17405.

[17] Dolghih, E.; Ortiz, W.; Kim, S.; Krueger, B. P.; Krause, J. L.; Roitberg, A. E. *J. Phys. Chem. A* 2009, 113, 4639-4646.

[18] Tanaka, S.; Scheraga, H. A. *Macromolecules* 1975, 8, 623-631.

[19] Vila, J. A.; Baldoni, H. A.; Ripoll, D. R.; Ghosh, A.; Scheraga, H. A. *Biophysical Journal* 2004, 86, 731-742.

[20] Reimer, U.; Scherer, G.; Drewello, M.; Kruber, S.; Schutkowski, M.; Fischer, G. *J. Mol. Biol.* 1998, 279, 449-460.

[21] Grathwohl, C.; Wuthrich, K. *Biopolymers* 1976, 15, 2025-2041.

[22] Grathwohl, C.; Wuthrich, K. *Biopolymers* 1976, 15, 2043-2057.

[23] Steinberg, I. Z.; Harrington, W. F.; Berger, A.; Sela, M.; Katchalski, E. *J. Am. Chem. Soc.* 1960, 82, 5263-5279.

[24] Gornick, F.; Mandelkern, L.; Diorio, A. F.; Roberts, D. E. *J. Am. Chem. Soc.* 1964, 86, 2549-2555.

[25] Mandelkern, L. *Poly-L-proline. In Poly-α-Amino Acids. G. D. Fasman, editor.;* Marcel Dekker: New York, 1967.

[26] Strassmair, H.; Engel, J.; Zundel, G. *Biopolymers* 1969, 8, 237-246.

[27] Tanaka, S.; Scheraga, H. A. *Macromolecules* 1975, 8, 504-516.

[28] Tanaka, S.; Scheraga, H. A. *Macromolecules* 1975, 8, 516-521.

[29] Kofron, J. L.; Kuzmic, P.; Kishore, V.; Colon-Bonilla, E.; Rich, D. H. *Biochemistry* 1991, 30, 6127-6134.

[30] Kakinoki, S.; Hirano, Y.; Oka, M. *Poly. Bul.* 2005, 53, 109-115.

[31] Traub, W.; Shmueli, U. *Nature* 1963, 198, 1165-1166.

[32] Cowan, P. M.; McGavin, S. *Nature* 1955, 176, 501-503.

[33] Mutter, M.; Wohr, T.; Gioria, S.; Keller, M. *Biopolymers* 1999, 51, 121-128.

[34] Tiffany, M. L.; Krimm, S. *Biopolymers* 1968, 6, 1379 – 1382.

[35] Tiffany, M. L.; Krimm, S. *Biopolymers* 1973, 12, 575 – 587.

[36] Shi, Z.; Olson, C. A.; Rose, G. D.; Baldwin, R. L.; Kallenbach, N. R. *Proc. Nat. Acad. Sci.* 2002, 99, 9190 – 9195.

[37] Shi, Z.; Woody, R. W.; Kallenbach, N. R. *Adv. Protein Chem.* 2002, 62, 163 – 240.

[38] Mohana-Borges, R.; Goto, N. K.; Kroon, G. J. A.; Dyson, H. J.; Wright, P. E. *J. Mol. Biol.* 2002, 340, 1131 – 1142.

[39] Keiderling, T. A.; Xu, Q. *Adv. Protein Chem.* 2002, 62, 91 – 162.

[40] Barron, L. D.; Blanch, E. W.; Hecht, L. *Adv. Protein Chem.* 2002, 62, 51 – 90.

[41] Mezei, M.; Fleming, P. J.; Srinivasan, R.; Rose, G. D. *PROTEINS* 2004, 55, 502 – 507.

[42] Graf, J.; Nguyen, P. H.; Stock, G.; Schwalbe, H. *JACS* 2007, 129, 1179 – 1189.

[43] Schweitzer-Stenner, R. *J. Phy. Chem. B* 2009, 113, 2922 – 2932.

[44] Duan, Y.; Wu, C.; Chowdhury, S.; Lee, M. C.; Xiong, G.; Zhang, W.; Yang, R.; Cieplak, P.; Luo, R.; Lee, T.; Caldwell, J.; Wang, J.; Kollman, P. *J. Comput. Chem.* 2003, 24, 1999 – 2012.

[45] Ferreon, J. C.; Hilser, V. J. *Prot. Sci.* 2003, 12, 982 – 996.

[46] Kohn, J. E.; Millett, I. S.; Jacob, J.; Zagrovic, B.; Dillon, T. M.; Cingel, N.; Dothager, R. S.; Seifert, S.; Thiyagarajan, P.; Sosnick, T. R.; Zahid Hasan, M.; Pande, V. S.; Ruczinski, I. Doniach, S.; Plaxco, K. W. *Proc. Nat. Acad. Sci.* 2004, 101, 12491 – 12496.

[47] McColl, I. H.; Blanch, E. W.; Hecht, L.; Kallenbach, N. R.; Barron, L. D. *J. Am. Chem. Soc* 2004, 126, 5076 – 5077.

[48] Vila, J. A.; Baldoni, H. A.; Ripoll, D. R.; Scheraga, H. A. *Proteins* 2004, 57, 87 – 98.

[49] Zagrovic, B.; Lipfert, J.; Sorin, E. J.; Millet, I. S.; van Gunsteren, W. F.; Doniach, S.; Pande, V. S. *Proc. Nat. Acad. Sci.* 2005, 102, 11698 – 11703.

[50] Makowska, J.; Rodziewicz-Motowidlo, S.; Baginska, K.; Vila, J. A.; Liwo, A.; Chumrzynski, L.; Scheraga, H. A. *Proc. Natl. Acad. Sci. USA.* 2006, 103, 1744-1749.

[51] Makowska, J.; Rodziewicz-Motowidlo, S.; Baginska, K.; Makowski, M.; Vila, J. A.; Liwo, A.; Chmurzynski, L.; Scheraga, H. A. *Biophysical Journal* 2007, 92, 2904 – 2917.

[52] Best, R. B.; Buchete, N.; Hummer, G. *Biophysical Journal: Biophysical Letters* 2008, 95, L07 – L09.

[53] Mukhopadhyaya, P.; Zubera, G.; Beratan, D. N. *Biophys. J.* 2008, 95, 5574 – 5586.

[54] Petrella, E. C.; Machesky, L. M.; Kaiser, D. A.; Pollard, T. D. *Biochemistry* 1996, 35, 16535 – 16543.

[55] Kelly, M. A.; Chellgren, B. W.; Rucker, A. L.; Troutman, J. M.; Fried, M. G.; Miller, A. F.; Creamer, T. P. *Biochemistry* 2001, 40, 14376-14383.

[56] Rucker, A. L.; Pager, C. T.; Campbell, M. N.; Qualls, J. E.; Creamer, T. P. *PROTEINS* 2003, 53, 68-75.

[57] Chellgren, B. W.; Creamer, T. P. *Biochemistry* 2004, 43, 5664 – 5669.

[58] Chellgren, B. W.; Creamer, T. P. *J. Am. Chem. Soc.* 2004, 126, 14734 – 14735.

[59] Whittington, S. J.; Chellgren, B. W.; Hermann, V. M.; Creamer, T. P. *Biochemistry* 2005, 44, 6269 – 6275.

[60] Chellgren, B. W.; Miller, A. F.; Creamer, T. P. *J. Mol. Biol.* 2006, 361, 362 – 371.

[61] Chakrabartty, A.; Kortemme, T.; Baldwin, R. L. *Protein Sci.* 1994, 3, 843 – 852.

[62] Lyu, P. C.; Liff, M. I.; Marky, L. A.; Kallenbach, N. R. *Science* 1990, 250, 669 – 673.

[63] Smith, C. K.; Withka, J. M. Regan, L. *Biochemistry* 1994, 33, 5510 – 5517.

[64] Minor, D. L.; Kim, P. S. *Nature* 1994, 371, 264 – 267.

[65] Ma, K.; Kan, L.; Wang, K. *Biochemistry* 2001, 40, 3427 – 3438.

[66] MacArthur, M. W.; Thornton, J. M. *J. Mol. Biol.* 1991, 218, 397 – 412.

[67] Grathwohl, C.; Wuthrich, K. *Biopolymers* 1981, 20, 2623-2633.

[68] Phillips, W. D. *J. Phys. Chem.* 1955, 23, 1363-1264.

[69] Pauling, L. *The Nature of the Chemical Bond, 3rd Ed.;* Cornell Univ. Press: Ithaca, NY, 1960.

[70] Tonelli, A. E. *J. Amer. Chem. Soc.* 1973, 95, 5946-5948.

[71] McDonald, D. C.; Still, W. C. *J. Org. Chem.* 1996, 61, 1385-1391.

[72] Venkatachalam, C. M.; Price, B. J.; Krimm, S. *Biopolymers* 2004, 14, 1121-1132.

[73] Kang, Y. K.; Choi, H. Y. *Biophysical Chemistry* 2004, 111, 135-142.

[74] Kang, Y. K.; Jhon, J. S.; Park, H. S. *J. Phys. Chem. B* 2006, 110, 17645-17655.

[75] Babin, V.; Roland, C.; Sagui, C. *J. Chem. Phys.* 2008, 128, 134101.

[76] Izrailev, S.; Stepaniants, Sand Isralewitz, B.; Kosztin, D.; Lu, H.; Molnar, F.; Wriggers, W.; Schulten, K. *Steered molecular dynamics. Computational Molecular Dynamics: Challenges, Methods, Ideas;* Springer-Verlag: Berlin, Germany, 1998.

[77] Geyer, C. J. Markov chain Monte Carlo maximum likelihood. In *Computing Science and Statistics: The 23rd symposium on the interface*; Interface Foundation: Fairfax, 1991.

[78] Huber, T.; Torda, A. E.; van Gunsteren, W. F. *J. Comput. Aided. Mol. Des.* 1994, 8, 695–708.

[79] Darve, E.; Pohorille, A. *J. Chem. Phys.* 2001, 115, 9169 – 9183.

[80] Wang, F.; Landau, D. P. *Phys. Rev. Lett.* 2001, 115, 2050 – 2053.

[81] Laio, A.; Parrinello, M. *Proc. Natl. Acad. Sci.* 2002, 99, 12562 – 12566.

[82] Iannuzzi, M.; Laio, A.; Parrinello, M. *Phys. Rev. Lett.* 2003, 90, 238302 – 1.

[83] Lelievre, T.; Rousset, M.; Stoltz, G. *J. Chem. Phys.* 2007, 126, 134111.

[84] Bussi, G.; Laio, A.; Parrinello, M. *Phys. Rev. Lett.* 2006, 96, 090601.

[85] Case, D. A. *et al.* *"AMBER 10";* University of California: San Francisco, 2008.

[86] Raiteri, P.; Laio, A.; Gervasio, F. L.; Micheletti, C.; Parrinello, M. *J. Phys. Chem.* 2006, 110, 3533 – 3539.

[87] Sugita, Y.; Kitao, A.; Okamoto, Y. *J. Chem. Phys.* 2000, 113, 6042.

[88] Babin, V.; Roland, C.; Darden, T. A.; Sagui, C. *J. Chem. Phys.* 2006, 125, 2049096.

[89] Babin, V.; Karpusenka, V.; Moradi, M.; Roland, C.; Sagui, C. *Int. J. of Q. Chem.* 2009, 109, 3666-3678.

[90] Babin, V.; Sagui, C. *J. Chem. Phys.* 2010, 132, 104108.

[91] Jarzynski, C. *Phys. Rev. Lett.* 1997, 78, 2690-2693.

[92] Crooks, G. E. *Phys. Rev. E* 2000, 61, 2361–2366.

[93] Shirts, M. R.; Bair, E.; Hooker, G.; Pande, V. y. S. *Phys. Rev. Lett.* 2003, 91, 140601.

[94] Kosztin, I.; Barz, B.; Janosi, L. *J. Chem. Phys.* 2006, 124, 064106.

[95] Laghaei, R.; Mousseau, N.; Wei, G. *J. Phys. Chem. B* 2010, 114, 7071-7077.

[96] Momany, F. A.; McGulre, R. F.; Burgess, A. W.; Scheraga, H. A. *J. Phys. Chem.* 1975, 79, 2361-2381.

[97] Madison, V. *Biopolymers* 1977, 16, 2671-2692.

[98] Vitagliano, L.; Berisio, R.; Mastrangelo, A.; Mazzarella, L.; Zagari, A. *Protein Sci.* 2001, 10, 2627-2632.

[99] Kang, Y. K. *J. Phys. Chem. B* 2007, 111, 10550-10556.

[100] Zimmerman, S. S.; Pottle, M. S.; Némethy, G.; Scheraga, H. A. *Macromolecules* 1977, 10, 1-9.

[101] Ramachandran, G. N.; Ramakrishnan, C.; Sasisekharan, V. *J. Mol. Biol.* 1963, 7, 95 – 99.

[102] Buhmann, J. M. Stochastic Algorithms For Exploratory Data Analysis: Data Clustering And Data Visualization. In *Learning in Graphical Models*; Kluwer: 1998.

[103] MacQueen, J. Some methods for classification and analysis of multivariate observations. In *Proceedings of the Fifth Berkeley Symposium on Mathematical Statistics and Probability, Volume 1: Statistics.*; Univ. of Calif. Press: 1967.

[104] Edwards, A. W. F. *Journal of the Royal Statistical Society. Series A (General)* 1963, 126, 109–114.

[105] Hawkins, G. D.; Cramer, C. J.; Truhlar, D. G. *J. Phys. Chem.* 1996, 100, 19824 – 39.

[106] Hawkins, G. D.; Cramer, C. J.; Truhlar, D. G. *Chem. Phys. Lett.* 1995, 246, 122 – 129.

[107] Tsui, V.; Case, D. A. *Biopolymers (Nucl. Acid. Sci.)* 2001, 56, 275-291.

[108] Cornell, W. D.; Cieplak, P.; Bayly, C. I.; Gould, I. R.; Merz, K. M.; Ferguson, D. M.; Spellmeyer, D. C.; Fox, T.; Caldwell, J. W.; Kollman, P. A. *J. Am. Chem. Soc.* 1995, 117, 5179 – 5197.

[109] Doshi, U.; Hamelberg, D. *J. Phys. Chem. B* 2009, 113, 16590 – 16595.

[110] Lin, L. N.; Brandts, J. F. *Biochemistry* 1979, 18, 5037-5042.

[111] Lin, L. N.; Brandts, J. F. *Biochemistry* 1980, 19, 3055-3059.

[112] Torchia, D. A.; Bovey, F. A. *Macromolecules* 1971, 4, 246-251.

[113] Creamer, T. P. *Proteins* 1998, 33, 218 – 226.

In: Proline
Editor: Bouzid Nedjimi

ISBN: 978-1-62257-739-2

Chapter VI

Central Functions of Proline in Behavior of Neonatal Chicks

Mitsuhiro Furuse[a], **Kousuke Hamasu**[a] and **D. Michael Denbow**[b]*

[a] Laboratory of Regulation in Metabolism and Behavior, Faculty of Agriculture, Kyushu University, Fukuoka, Japan

[b] Department of Animal and Poultry Sciences, Virginia Tech, Blacksburg, VA, US

Abstract

Proline is formally an imino acid, but is usually called an amino acid. It is not an essential amino acid, since proline is biosynthetically derived from the amino acid L-glutamate. Food intake was mildly stimulated by low levels of intracerebroventricular (i.c.v.) injection of L-proline, but was suppressed by high levels in chicks. L-Proline was decreased in the telencephalon and diencephalon under several different stressors including restraint with isolation-induced and fasting stress. Central L-proline induced sedative and hypnotic effects in a dose-dependent manner, suggesting that L-proline may

* Correspondence to: Mitsuhiro Furuse, Laboratory of Regulation in Metabolism and Behavior, Faculty of Agriculture, Kyushu University, Fukuoka 812-8511, Japan, Tel/Fax: (81) (92) 642-2953, E-mail: furuse@brs.kyushu-u.ac.jp

have an important role in attenuating the stress response in the central nervous system of chicks.

The central effects of L-proline, D-proline and *trans*-4-hydroxy-L-proline were investigated by using the acute stressful model with neonatal chicks. Sedative and hypnotic effects were induced by all compounds, while plasma corticosterone release under isolation stress was only attenuated by L-proline. To clarify the mechanism by which L-proline and D-proline induce sedative and hypnotic effects, the contribution of the strychnine-sensitive glycine receptor (glycine receptor) and *N*-methyl-D-aspartate glutamate receptor (NMDA receptor) were further investigated. The glycine receptor antagonist strychnine was co-injected i.c.v. with L-proline or D-proline. The suppression of isolation-induced stress behavior by D-proline was attenuated by strychnine. However, the suppression of stress behavior by L-proline was not attenuated. The NMDA receptor antagonist (+)-MK-801 was co-injected i.c.v. with L-proline. The suppression of stress behavior by L-proline was attenuated by (+)-MK-801. These results indicate that L-proline and D-proline differentially induce sedative and hypnotic effects through NMDA and glycine receptors, respectively. Using microdialysis, the effect of L-proline on monoamine release in the medio-rostral neostriatum/hyperstriatum ventrale (MNH) of freely moving and restricted chicks was investigated. A 30 min handling stress resulted in significant increases of extracellular homovallinic acids (HVA), a dopamine metabolite, and 5-hydroxyindoleacetic acid (5-HIAA), a serotonin metabolite, in the MNH. L-Proline, perfused through a microdialysis probe in the MNH during the stressed condition, significantly attenuated the average dialysate concentration of HVA produced by handling-stress. Handling-stress resulted in a significant increase in 5-HIAA levels in the control group, which were attenuated by profusion with L-proline. These results show that perfusion of L-proline decreased the release of dopamine and serotonin in the MNH caused by handling-stress.

1. Introduction

L-Proline (abbreviated as Pro or P) is formally an imino acid (Fig. 1), but is usually treated as one of the twenty DNA-encoded α-amino acids. Its codons are CCU, CCC, CCA, and CCG. It is not a nutritionally essential amino acid, which means that the animal body can synthesize it from L-glutamate. First, the γ-carboxyl group of L-glutamate reacts with ATP to form an acyl phosphate. This mixed anhydride is then reduced by NADPH to an aldehyde. Glutamic γ-semialdehyde forms a ring structure with a loss of H_2O in a nonenzymatic process to give Δ^1-pyrroline-5-carboxylate, which is reduced by NADPH to L-Pro.

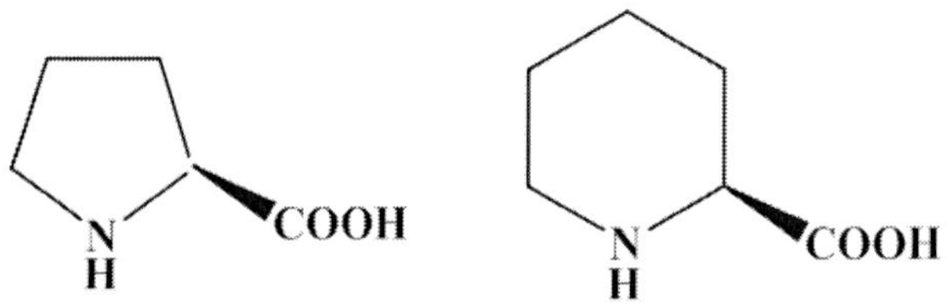

L-Proline (L-Pro) **L-Homoproline (L-Pipecolic acid, L-PA)**

Figure 1. Structures of L-proline and L-homoproline.

L-Pro also has an aliphatic side chain, but it differs from other amino acids in that its side chain is bonded to both the nitrogen and the α-carbon atoms. L-Pro markedly influences protein architecture because L-Pro is the only amino acid that contains a cyclized substituted α-amino group and its ring structure makes it more conformationally restricted than the other amino acids. L-Pro is very rigid, and its presence creates a fixed kink in a protein chain. L-Pro is sometimes found at points on a protein's surface where the chain loops back into the protein. The presence of a built-in bend, in the case of L-Pro, allows the polypeptide backbone to fold into a tight U-shaped structure. L-Pro is usually found in the triple-helical structure of collagen, since it arises from an unusual abundance of three amino acids: glycine (Gly), L-Pro, and hydroxyproline. These amino acids make up the characteristic repeating motif Gly-Pro-X, where X can be any amino acid. Each amino acid has a precise function. The fixed angle of the C-N peptidyl-proline or peptidyl-hydroxyproline bond enables each polypeptide chain to fold into a helix with a geometry such that three polypeptide chains can twist together to form a three-stranded helix. Interestingly, although the rigid peptidyl-proline linkages disrupt the packing of amino acids in an α helix, they stabilize the rigid three-stranded collagen helix. L-Pro is also involved in numerous physiologic processes including glucogenesis and lipogenesis (Sugden et al., 1984, Baquet et al., 1991).

The amino acids that can activate the Gly receptor include β-alanine, taurine, L-alanine, L-serine and L-Pro. γ-Aminobutyric acid (GABA) is inactive at this receptor. However, L-homoproline (L-pipecolic acid, L-PA), which contains a methylene group added to L-Pro (Fig. 1) and is synthesized as a major metabolic intermediate of L-lysine in the brain, may influence the GABAergic system. In behavioral tests, the intracerebroventricular (i.c.v.) injection of L-PA reduced active wakefulness and feeding behavior while inducing sleep-like behavior. The role of the GABA-A or GABA-B receptors in the suppression of food intake and induction of sleep-like behavior by L-PA was investigated (Takagi et al., 2003a). Chicks were injected i.c.v. with L-PA and the GABA-A antagonist picrotoxin or GABA-B antagonist CGP54626. Although suppression of food intake by L-PA was partially attenuated by co-injection with CGP54626, but not picrotoxin, sleep-like behavior induced by L-PA was significantly suppressed by both antagonists. These results suggest that L-PA activated both GABA-A and GABA-B receptors, and that GABA-B receptors contributed to food intake while both receptors contributed to sleep-like behavior under fasting conditions.

These facts imply that not only L-PA, but also L-Pro, as a free form function in the central nervous system (CNS). Firstly, we discuss our study showing that central L-Pro modified food intake in neonatal chicks (Haraguchi et al., 2007). Secondly, we discuss the function of L-Pro under stressful conditions (Hamasu et al., 2009a). Thirdly, the mechanism by which L-Pro and D-Pro induced sedative and hypnotic effcts under an acute stress is examined (Hamasu et al., 2010). Then, involvement of cholinergic (Hamasu et al., 2009b) and monoaminergic systems (Hamasu et al., 2009c) are discussed.

2. I.C.V Injection of L-Pro Modifies Food Intake in Neonatal Chicks

According to one accepted classification, some amino acids are termed essential amino acids (sometimes called indispensable), meaning that they must be supplied via the diet. Nine amino acids (L-histidine, L-isoleucine, L-leucine, L-lysine, L-methionine, L-phenylalanine, L-threonine, L-tryptophan and L-valine) are generally regarded as essential for humans. The others, which used to be classified as nonessential, are now more correctly termed dispensable amino acids (L-alanine, L-aspartic acid, L-cystine, L-glutamic acid and L-serine) or conditionally indispensable (L-arginine, L-cysteine, Gly and L-tyrosine), meaning they are not normally required in the diet, but must be supplied exogenously to specific populations that do not synthesize it in adequate amounts. The central function of both dispensable and indispensable amino acids on behavior has been clarified. Those amino acids that can activate the Gly receptor including Gly (Asechi et al., 2006), β-alanine (Tomonaga et al., 2004), L-alanine (Kurauchi et al., 2006) and L-serine (Koutoku et al., 2005; Asechi et al., 2006) have been shown to have sedative and/or hypnotic effects.

L-PA, a major metabolic intermediate of L-lysine, is also an imine and has a unique function in the brain for the regulation of food intake. Under fasting conditions, central L-PA is an anorexigenic factor (Takagi et al., 2001, 2003a). However, it has the opposite effect under *ad libitum* feeding conditions in which brain injections of L-PA act as an orexigenic factor (Takagi et al., 2003b).

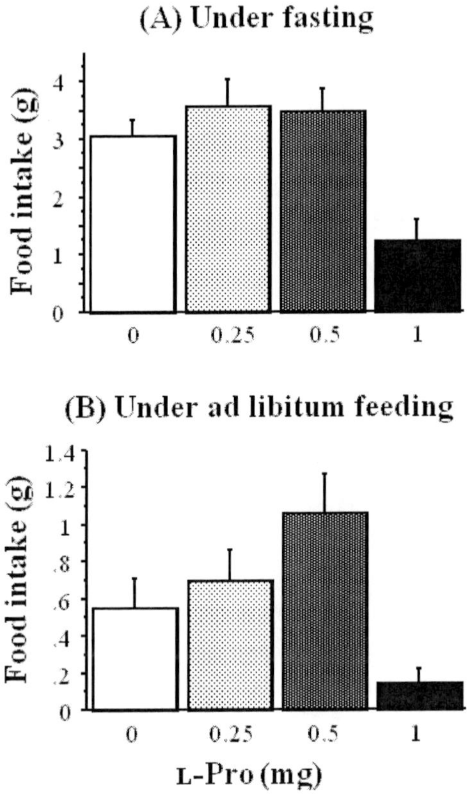

Figure 2. Effect of i.c.v. injection of L-Pro on food intake of chicks under (A) a fasting condition and (B) an ad libitum feeding condition. Data are expressed as means ± S.E.M. Reproduced from Haraguchi, T., Tomonaga, S., Kurauchi, I., Hamasu, K., Sato, H., Denbow, D.M. and Furuse, M., Intracerebroventricular injection of L-proline modifies food intake in neonatal chicks, J. Anim. Vet. Adv., 6(2007):1255-1257.

According to Davis et al. (1979), the i.c.v. injection of C^{14}-labeled L-Pro in neonatal chicks resulted in its distribution in periventricular tissue, including the septum, hippocampus, and hypothalamus, 1 min after injection. This fact suggests that i.c.v. injected L-Pro quickly distributes within the brain. This characteristic of L-Pro clearly reflected on food intake for 60 min after injection. Fig. 2(A) shows the effect of i.c.v. injection of L-Pro on 60 min food intake of chicks after food deprivation for 3 h. The following regression equation was obtained: food intake

(g) = 3.047 (SE 0.339) + 3.496 (SE 1.765)x – 5.332 (1.654)x^2 (x in mg of L-Pro, R^2=0.466, RMS=1.056) (Haraguchi et al., 2007). Food intake was mildly increased and then decreased severely in a dose dependent manner. The most efficacious dose of L-Pro under fasting conditions was calculated as 0.12 mg from the curve. Fig. 2(B) shows the effect of i.c.v. injection of L-Pro on 60 min food intake of chicks under an *ad libitum* feeding condition. The regression equation obtained was: food intake (g) = 0.479 (SE 0.164) + 2.130 (SE 0.815)x – 2.452 (0.747)x^2 (R^2=0.313, RMS=0.487) (Haraguchi et al., 2007). Under *ad libitum* conditions the most efficacious dose was 0.35 mg. These facts imply that the addition of small amounts of L-Pro to the diet may improve food intake. On the other hand, L-Pro does not cross the blood-brain barrier readily (Davis et al., 1979), therefore, the dietary effect of L-Pro on food intake remains to be determined.

The response of L-Pro under *ad libitum* feeding conditions was somewhat different from the effect of L-PA, since central administration of L-PA enhanced food intake at i.c.v. levels of 0.5 and 1 mg (Takagi et al., 2003b). The response under fasting conditions was similar between L-Pro and L-PA (Takagi et al., 2001, 2003a) in that 1 mg of both L-Pro (Haraguchi et al., 2007) and L-PA (Takagi et al., 2001, 2003a) severely suppressed food intake.

While we hypothesized that imines such as L-Pro and L-PA would have a similar function on feeding, it appears that their functions are different depending on the feeding conditions. The difference may be explained by the following reason. Takagi et al. (2003a, b) revealed that L-PA worked through GABA receptors whereas L-Pro binds to Gly receptor as well as glutamate receptors (Henzi et al., 1992). Later, it was clear that the *N*-methyl-D-aspartate (NMDA) glutamate receptor was associated with the function of L-Pro, but not Gly receptor, in neonatal chicks (Hamasu et al., 2010). This will be discussed in the fourth section. The difference in the receptor may influence food intake. In conclusion, L-Pro can act in the chick brain to modulate food intake, its effect being dependent on the dose.

3. L-Pro is A Sedative Regulator of Acute Stress in the Brain of Neonatal Chicks

In the CNS, some amino acids have very important functions as neurotransmitters. In particular, the roles of L-glutamate and GABA in the stress response have received much attention. Knowledge of the involvement of amino acids in neural regulation is still expanding (Boehning and Snyder, 2003). For example, sedative and hypnotic effects of some amino acids such as L-serine, L-cysteine, Gly (Asechi et al., 2006), L-alanine (Kurauchi et al., 2006), L-arginine (Suenaga et al., 2008a), L-ornithine (Suenaga et al., 2008b) and β-alanine (Tomonaga et al., 2004) under an acute stressful condition were reported in neonatal chicks. However, these results were obtained using exogenous amino acid adminstration, since the responses were confirmed by i.c.v. injection of amino acids. Therefore, whether or not endogenous amino acid metabolism in the brain is affected by stress was still unclear.

Previously, the behaviors of chicks were investigated under stressful conditions (Panksepp et al., 1980b, Sahley et al., 1981, Feltenstein et al., 2003). For instance, chicks feel comfortable when they are in crowds, but feel acute stress when they are isolated. The isolation-induced stress increases spontaneous activity and vocalization. This isolation–induced stress paradigm has been used to objectively screen anxiolytic drugs, measuring vocalization and spontaneous activity as the index of behaviors induced by stressor.

A survey of amino acids which are rapidly metabolized under stressful conditions was conducted, since such amino acids are required to attenuate stress responses in the brain. Under restraint with isolation-induced stress, L-glutamine was significantly higher, whereas GABA, L-arginine, and L-Pro were significantly lower than those of the control group in the telencephalon (Hamasu et al., 2009a). In the diencephalon, L-alanine, L-arginine, L-asparagine, L-aspartic acid, L-phenylalanine, L-Pro, L-serine, and L-tyrosine were significantly lower following restraint with isolation-induced stress than those of the control group. Under fasting stress, on the other hand, L-tyrosine and L-valine were significantly increased at 6 h after fasting, whereas L-arginine, L-histidine, and L-Pro were significantly decreased after 3 h fasting compared with the control group in the telencephalon (Hamasu et al., 2009a). In the diencephalon, L-tyrosine was significantly increased at 6 h fasting, whereas L-arginine, L-asparagine, L-aspartic acid, L-glutamine, L-histidine, L-phenylalanine, and L-Pro were significantly decreased after 3 h fasting compared to the control group. It was clear that the contents of several amino acids were modified under stressful conditions and the response of amino acids during stress was mainly a reduction in their contents. Among amino acids modified, L-arginine and L-Pro were reduced in both the telencephalon and diencephalon under both restraint with isolation-induced stress and fasting stresses. Both amino acids may be rapidly metabolized in the brain under stressful conditions. For L-arginine, Suenaga et al. (2008a) reported that central L-arginine functions to attenuate stress responses. Furthermore, the mechanism of sedation induced by L-arginine was revealed by the same group.

The sedative effect of L-arginine was mainly mediated by L-ornithine and by cooperation with other free amino acids having sedative and hypnotic effects in the CNS (Suenaga et al., 2008b). L-Ornithine is a metabolite of L-arginine. L-Arginine might be converted to L-ornithine for sedative and hypnotic effects under stressful conditions. Therefore, brain L-arginine of the stress groups was significantly lower than in the control group. Central functions of L-arginine and its metabolites for stress behavior have already been reviewed by Tomonaga et al. (2011). Later, Kurata et al. (2011) revealed that L-ornithine functions through GABA-A receptors.

The effects of L-Pro on various physiologic activities have been reported in past studies. For example, it produces a depressor response when microinjected into the caudal ventrolateral medulla of anesthetized rats (Takemoto et al., 2005). However, the function of L-Pro during the stress response had not been investigated. Therefore, the i.c.v. injection of L-Pro examined whether centrally administered L-Pro could modify the behavior of neonatal chicks under isolation-induced stress (Hamasu et al., 2009a). When the effect of i.c.v. injection of several doses of L-Pro on spontaneous activity and distress vocalizations during the 10 min isolation-induced stress was determined, negative correlations between the dose of L-Pro and spontaneous activity and total distress vocalization were detected. Based on the method by van Luijtelaar et al. (1987), the behaviors were classified into four categories: (1) active wakefulness; (2) standing/sitting motionless with eyes opened; (3) standing motionless with eyes closed; and (4) sitting motionless with head drooped (sleeping posture) by watching videotapes. van Luijtelaar et al. (1987) demonstrated the correlation between sleeping posture and electrophysiological sleep with EEG measurement. The time for active wakefulness was reduced with increasing dose of L-Pro. Negative correlations between the dose of L-Pro and the time for active wakefulness were detected. Additionally, L-Pro increased the time for standing or sitting motionless with eyes open and sleeping posture. These results revealed the novel function that L-Pro has sedative and hypnotic effects under an acute stressful condition in neonatal chicks.

These effects of i.c.v. L-Pro may have a considerable link to several mechanisms of neurotransmission in the CNS. L-Pro has been suggested as a neuronal modulator or transmitter candidate in the CNS for many years (Snyder et al., 1973). In addition, Henzi et al. (1992) revealed that L-Pro binds to Gly and glutamate receptors. Gly (Asechi et al., 2006) and L-glutamate (Yamane et al., 2009) cause a sedative and hypnotic effect, as observed with L-Pro. So, the sedative and hypnotic effects of L-Pro were possibly associated with the modulation of these receptor functions in the brain. These possibilities are clarified in the fourth section. Secondly, metabolites of L-Pro might be responsible for sedative and hypnotic effects. L-Pro metabolism involves two other amino acids, L-glutamate and L-ornithine. This tri-amino acid system also links with three other essential metabolic systems, the TCA cycle, urea cycle, and pentose phosphate pathway (Hu et al., 2008). Namely, L-Pro and its metabolites might affect these pathways and induce sedative and hypnotic effects.

In conclusion, L-Pro was significantly decreased in the telencephalon and diencephalon of neonatal chicks when several types of stress were applied. Furthermore, the i.c.v. injection of L-Pro had sedative and hypnotic effects under an acute stressful condition in neonatal chicks. From these results, it is expected that L-Pro might improve anxiety disorders or sleep disorders induced by a stressor.

4. I.C.V Injection of L-Pro and D-Pro Induces Sedative and Hypnotic Effects by Different Mechanisms under an Acute Stressful Condition in Chicks

There are many studies suggesting that L-Pro may be a neuronal modulator or transmitter candidate in the CNS (Snyder et al., 1973; Yoneda and Roberts, 1982; Fremeau et al., 1992; Gogos et al., 1999; Renick et al., 1999). As mentioned above, the amount of L-Pro in the brain was reduced under stressful conditions, and i.c.v. injection of L-Pro had sedative and hypnotic effects under an acute stressful condition in neonatal chicks (Hamasu et al., 2009a). From these facts, it appears that L-Pro might function through several neurotransmitter systems in the CNS. However, the mechanism by which L-Pro attenuates stress behavior has not been clarified with special reference to proline-related compounds such as D-Pro and *trans*-4-hydroxy- L-Pro under the acute stressful model in neonatal chicks. All L-Pro, D-Pro, and *trans*-4-hydroxy-L-Pro significantly decreased distress vocalizations compared to the control. D-Pro and *trans*-4-hydroxy-L-Pro had no effect on plasma corticosterone levels. L-Pro, D-Pro, and *trans*-4-hydroxy-L-Pro induced sedative and hypnotic effects compared with the saline control. However, only L-Pro significantly lowered the plasma corticosterone level compared to the control group, and these values were as low as that of the intact group in which chicks were housed in groups. Therefore, L-Pro might have the ability to directly suppress the secretion of corticosterone from the adrenal glands through the hypothalamic-pituitary-adrenal (HPA) axis in response to stress. On the other hand, D-Pro and *trans*-4-hydroxy-L-Pro appear not to have such an effect. As a result, the mechanism of sedative and hypnotic effects of L-Pro in chicks appears different from D-Pro and *trans*-4-hydroxy-L-Pro.

Therefore, the receptors that mediate the actions of these compounds were obscure and the mechanism of L-Pro and D-Pro was further examined. The strychnine-sensitive Gly receptor is a pentameric ligand-gated anion channel composed of two different subunits, α and β. Also, the NMDA glutamate receptor is an excitatory amino acid ligand-gated ion channel that is selectively activated by NMDA and regulated at several pharmacologically distinct sites. This receptor is present in both the hypothalamus (Halpain et al., 1984) and pituitary (Lindstrom and Ohlsson, 1992), suggesting its role in neuroendocrine regulation (Mahesh et al., 1999). Past studies showed that although L- and D-Pro can activate the Gly receptor, the NMDA receptor is activated by L-Pro alone (Henzi et al. 1992; Ortiz et al. 1996). In addition, Gly (Asechi et al., 2006) and L-glutamate (Yamane et al., 2009) caused a sedative and hypnotic effect similar to that observed with L-Pro. So, it was hypothesized that these receptors are involved in the action of proline to induce sedative and hypnotic effects. To clarify these possibilities, the Gly receptor antagonist, strychnine, and NMDA receptor antagonist, (+)-MK-801, were applied (Hamasu et al., 2010). The effect of L-Pro on distress vocalization and behavioral changes could not be attenuated by strychnine. On the other hand, the suppressive effect of D-Pro on distress-induced vocalizations was moderately attenuated by co-injection of strychnine. D-Pro increased sitting motionless with head drooped (sleeping posture) and decreased active wakefulness, and strychnine attenuated these effects. Sleeping posture induced by D-Pro was attenuated by co-injection with strychnine and consequently, the behavior of chicks tended toward wakefulness (Hamasu et al., 2010). These results indicate that the Gly receptor is involved in sedative and hypnotic effects induced by D-Pro, but not L-Pro. *In vitro*, L-Pro can activate the Gly receptor (Henzi et al., 1992; Ortiz et al., 1996). However, this receptor is not involved in the action of L-Pro to induce sedative and hypnotic effects.

The suppressive effect of L-Pro on distress-induced vocalizations was attenuated by co-injection of (+)-MK801 (Hamasu et al., 2010). Sleeping posture induced by L-Pro was attenuated by co-injection with (+)-MK801 and consequently, the behavior of chicks tended toward wakefulness. The NMDA receptor is well established as playing important roles in neuroendocrine regulation (Mahesh et al., 1999). In fact, NMDA stimulates corticotrophin-releasing hormone release from rat hypothalamic slices, and this effect is inhibited by an NMDA receptor antagonist (Joanny et al., 1997). Several studies examined the role of the NMDA receptor *in vivo*. Systemic administration of NMDA enhanced adrenocorticotropin (ACTH) and serum corticosterone secretion (Farah et al., 1991), and the secretion of ACTH in response to immobilization stress was inhibited by a NMDA centrally acting receptor antagonist (Jezová et al., 1995). Thus, this receptor is involved in the regulation of the HPA axis. The increase in plasma corticosterone induced by isolation stress was suppressed with i.c.v. injections of L-Pro. Presumably, this effect was mediated via the NMDA receptor activity which was modulated by L-Pro. Previous studies indicated that activation of dopaminergic and serotonergic pathways are related to behavioral and emotional changes (Abercrombie et al., 1989; Gruss et al., 1996). For example, isolation-induced stress resulted in a significant increase of 5-hydroxyindoleacetic acid and only a slight increase of homovanillic acid in the forebrain of domestic chicks (Gruss et al., 1996). Additionally, some experiments suggested a modulatory interaction between the glutamatergic and monoaminergic pathway, which is mediated via NMDA receptor activation (Gruss et al., 1999). Arco and Mora (2001) showed that local activation of prefrontal NMDA receptors reduced the stress-induced dopamine release in the prefrontal cortex of the rat. From these findings, we assumed that L-Pro modulates activation of NMDA receptors and alters activation of dopaminergic and serotonergic pathways. Through this mechanism, i.c.v. injection of L-Pro might induce sedative and hypnotic effects under an acute stressful condition in neonatal chicks. Indeed, i.c.v. injection of L-Pro suppressed the increase in serotonin turnover rate and slightly suppressed the increase in dopamine turnover rate induced by isolation stress in the telencephalon (Hamasu et al., 2012). In conclusion, the i.c.v. injection of L-Pro and D-Pro induces sedative and hypnotic effects under an acute stressful condition in neonatal chicks. However, L-Pro, but not D-Pro, significantly lowered plasma corticosterone level. Probably, it is attributed to a difference in the mechanism of action. The mechanism of attenuation of the acute stress response by L-Pro is mediated by the modulation of the NMDA receptor in the CNS. On the contrary, D-Pro is mediated by the modulation of the glycine receptor.

5. Cholinergic Neurotransmission Is Not Involved in Sedation Induced by L-Pro in Neonatal Chicks

Numerous studies have shown that the cholinergic systems are involved in emotionally guided behavior. For example, there is evidence that acetylcholine

(ACh) receptor (AChR) antagonists increase fear reactions (Hess and Blozovski, 1987; Smythe et al., 1998), whereas increasing cholinergic activity reduced fear reactions (Degroot and Parent, 2001; Degroot et al., 2001). In addition, hippocampal cholinergic blockade enhanced the HPA response to stress (Bhatnagar et al., 1997). These facts indicate that the hippocampal cholinergic system regulates stress-induced HPA activity and serves to coordinate behavioral responses to stress. Furthermore, the cholinergic systems play an important role in the stress response of chicks in which AChR agonists decreased isolation stress-induced vocalizations while antagonists had the opposite effect (Panksepp et al., 1980a, Sahley et al., 1981).

ACh esterase (AChE) plays a key role in cholinergic transmission in the CNS, terminating the synaptic action of ACh. Delwing et al. (2003) showed that L-Pro has an inhibitory effect of AChE in the brain suggesting that L-Pro increases synaptic ACh levels and facilitates cholinergic activity.

A previous study has shown that i.c.v. injection of L-Pro induces sedative effects in neonatal chicks mediated by the NMDA receptor under an acute stressful condition (Hamasu et al., 2010).

It was predicted that the cholinergic systems might also be involved in the effect of L-Pro. In chicks, the AChR plays an important role in the control of separation stress-induced vocalization. Non-selective AChR agonists decreased isolation stress-induced vocalization while antagonists had the opposite effect (Panksepp et al., 1980a, b). The AChR has two subtypes, M-AChR and nicotinic AChR (N-AChR). Sahley et al. (1981) suggested that M-AChR was involved in controlling vocalizations more than the N-AChR. To examine whether the sedative effects of L-Pro are associated with modulation of cholinergic neurotransmission, L-Pro was co-injected with the M-AChR antagonist scopolamine to determine the effects on the behavior of neonatal chicks under isolation-induced stress (Hamasu et al., 2009c). Fig. 3 shows the effect of i.c.v. injection of L-Pro with or without scopolamine on spontaneous activity (upper panel) and distress vocalizations (lower panel) during the 10 min isolation-induced stress. L-Pro significantly decreased spontaneous activity and the number of vocalizations.

However, no significant effects of scopolamine were observed in spontaneous activity or the number of vocalizations. Interactions between L-Pro and scopolamine were not detected in either spontaneous activity or the number of vocalizations. These results imply that the effect of L-Pro could not be attenuated by scopolamine. Therefore, the M-AChR does not appear to be involved in the sedative effects induced by L-Pro.

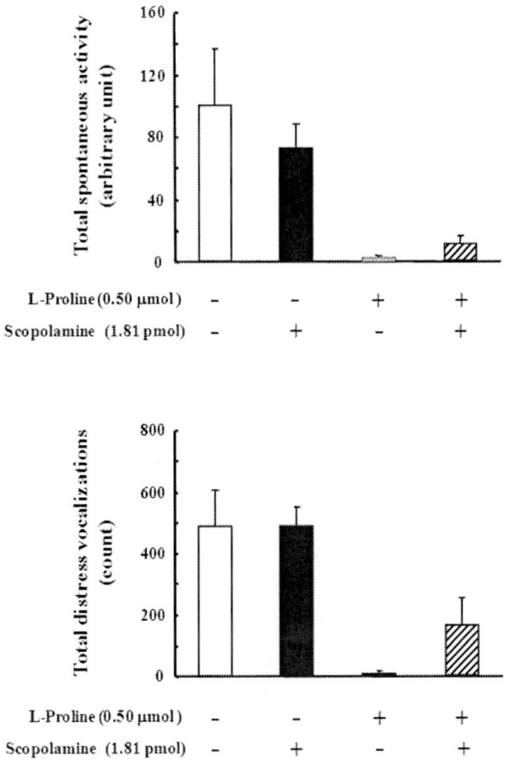

Figure 3. Effect of i.c.v. injection of either 1.81 pmol of scopolamine, 0.50 μmol of L-Pro, or scopolamine plus L-Pro on total spontaneous activity (upper panel) and distress vocalizations (lower panel) during 10 min isolation in 4- or 5-day-old layer chicks. Results are expressed as means±S.E.M. Reproduced from Hamasu, K., Shigemi, K., Tsuneyoshi, Y., Sato, H., Denbow, D.M. and Furuse, M., Cholinergic neurotransmission is not involved in sedation induced by L-proline in neonatal chicks. J. Anim. Vet. Adv., 8(2009c):1207-1211.

Delwing et al. (2003) showed that L-Pro reduces AChE activity in the cerebral cortex of rats. The AChE activity was significantly decreased in the rat brain following a single s.c. injection of L-Pro. Furthermore, L-Pro also inhibited AChE activity *in vitro*. The effect of i.c.v. injection of several doses of L-Pro on AChE activity in the telencephalon and diencephalon of chicks was investigated (Hamasu et al., 2009c). L-Pro had no significant effect on either telencephalon or diencephalon AChE activity. These results differed from those by Delwing et al. (2003). Hamasu et al. (2009c) injected L-Pro directly to the lateral ventricle, while Delwing et al. (2003) injected s.c. Accordingly, some peripheral routes might be involved in brain AChE activities. Furthermore, these varying results might be attributed to the concentration of L-Pro, interval of time after injection, effect of isolation stress, or species differences.

The results obtained here indicate that the cholinergic systems are not involved in the sedative effects induced by L-Pro.

6. Central L-Pro Attenuates Stress-Induced Dopamine and Serotonin Metabolism in the Chick Forebrain

While L-glutamate is well established as a neurotransmitter in the CNS, little is known about the possible role of L-Pro as a neurotransmitter. The amount of L-Pro in the brain was reduced under stressful conditions, and i.c.v. injection of L-Pro had sedative and hypnotic effects under an acute stressful condition in neonatal chicks (Hamasu et al., 2009a). Therefore, it appears that L-Pro might function through several neurotransmitter systems in the CNS. Past studies showed that L-Pro can activate the strychnine-sensitive Gly receptor and the NMDA glutamate receptor (David et al., 1992; Henzi et al., 1992; Ortiz et al., 1996, Cohen and Nadler, 1997). The NMDA, but not Gly, receptor appears involved in the action of L-Pro to induce sedative and hypnotic effects (Hamasu et al., 2010).

Activation of dopaminergic and serotonergic pathways are related to behavioral and emotional changes (Abercrombie et al., 1989; Gruss and Braun, 1997). Some experiments suggested a modulatory interaction between the glutamatergic and monoaminergic pathway, which is mediated via NMDA receptor activation (Jedema and Moghaddam, 1996, Gruss et al., 1999). From these findings, we assumed that L-Pro activates the NMDA receptor and alters activation of dopaminergic and serotonergic pathways. Indeed, i.c.v. injection of L-Pro suppressed the increase in serotonin turnover rate and slightly suppressed the increase in dopamine turnover rate induced by isolation stress in the telencephalon (Hamasu et al., 2012). However, the effect of L-Pro on the release of stress-induced monoamines is still obscure. Hamasu et al. (2009b) investigated the interaction of L-Pro and monoamine release in the medio-rostral neostriatum/hyperstriatum ventrale (MNH) during stress. The MNH, a presumed analogue of the mammalian prefrontal cortex (Metzger et al., 1996, 2002), was identified to be involved in the stress response (Gruss and Braun, 1997, Muller and Scheich, 1986). Hamasu et al. (2009b) determined dialysate concentrations of homovallinic acids (HVA), a dopamine (DA) metabolite, and 5-

hydroxyindoleacetic acid (5-HIAA), a serotonin (5-HT) metabolite. In their study, DA and 5-HT were not detectable, due to low concentrations, but their metabolites, HVA and 5-HIAA, were clearly detected. These metabolites may, at least in part, reflect release of their respective neurotransmitters (Gruss and Braun, 1997; Gruss et al., 1999).

Fig. 4 shows the effects of L-Pro (100 mM) on stress-stimulated dialysate concentrations of HVA (upper panel) and 5-HIAA (lower panel). There was a significant interaction between the control and L-Pro group on HVA, suggesting that L-Pro significantly reduced the average increases of dialysate concentration of HVA produced by handling-stress. In contrast, there was no significant interaction in 5-HIAA. However, the 30 min handling-stress resulted in a significant increase in 5-HIAA levels in the control group, while there was no increase in the L-Pro group.

The results demonstrated that the increases of dialysate concentration of HVA and 5-HIAA in the MNH caused by handling-stress were attenuated by the simultaneous perfusion of L-Pro (100 mM). It is suggested that these effects of L-Pro were mediated by the NMDA receptor, given that a previous study indicated that L-Pro modulated activation of the NMDA receptor (Hamasu et al., 2010). The microdialysis study by Gruss et al. (1999) which showed a modulatory interaction between glutamatergic and monoaminergic neurotransmission mediated by the NMDA receptor further supports this suggestion. They demonstrated that the dialysate concentration of HVA and 5-HIAA were decreased by local intracerebral infusion of NMDA, and these effects were antagonized by an NMDA antagonist. However, no decrease was confirmed by local intracerebral infusion of L-Pro. The cause of this discrepancy may be the concentration of L-Pro. The dialysate concentration of HVA and 5-HIAA might be decreased by infusion of higher concentrations of L-Pro. Del Arco and Mora (2001) reported that NMDA (100 μM) significantly reduced the average increases of dialysate concentration of DA without modifying basal dialysate in DA.

Regarding the mechanisms of action, NMDA may stimulate GABAergic interneurons in the MNH region, which inhibit monoaminergic synaptic boutons and thereby reduce local neurotransmitter release. This suggestion is supported by studies in which endogenous glutamate increases GABA (Del Arco et al., 1999) and GABA agonists inhibit dopamine release in the prefrontal cortex (Doherty and Gratton, 1999; Santiago et al., 1993). Furthermore, L-PA has a similar structure to L-Pro, since it is an imino acid having a ring structure. According to Takagi et al. (2003a), L-PA activated both GABA-A and GABA-B receptors. L-Pro may also stimulate GABAergic interneurons and may reduce local transmitter release, so the increases of dialysate concentration of HVA and 5-HIAA in the MNH caused by handling-stress may be attenuated.

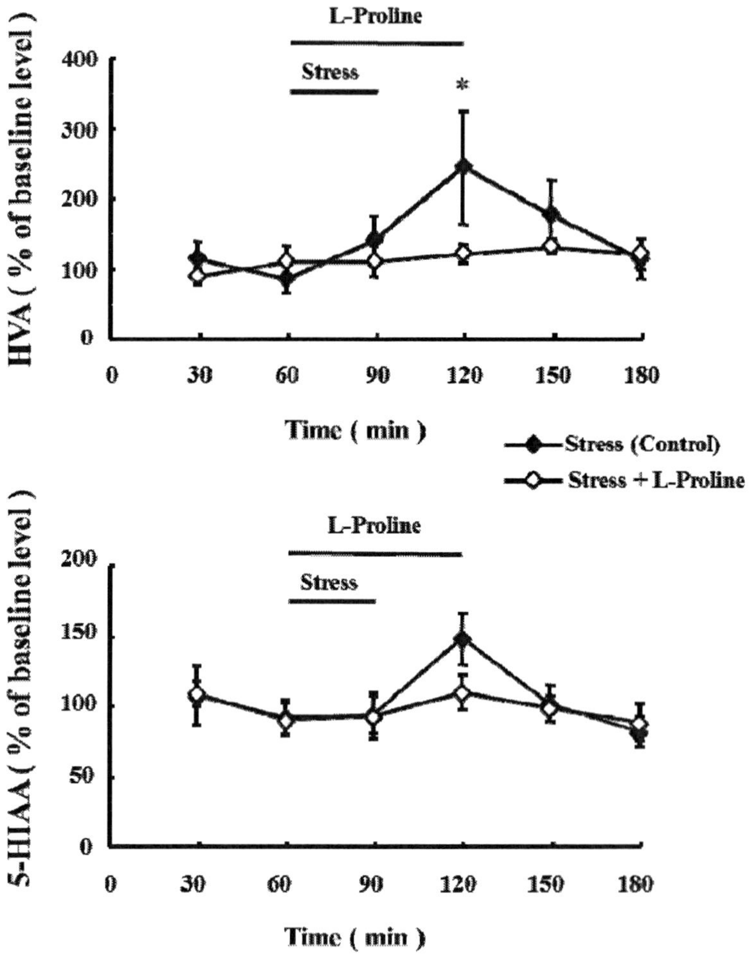

Figure 4. Effects of L-proline (100 mM), perfused through the microdialysis probe for 60 min, on increases of HVA and 5-HIAA produced by a 30 min handling-stress in the medio-rostral neostriatum/hyperstriatum ventrale (MNH) of awake 8- or 9-day-old layer chicks. Results are expressed as means±S.E.M. *, Significantly different from the data that was collected just before the beginning of stress. Reproduced from Hamasu, K., Shigemi, K., Kabuki, Y., Tomonaga, S., Denbow, D.M. and Furuse, M., Central L-proline attenuates stress-induced dopamine and serotonin metabolism in the chick forebrain, Neurosci. Lett., 460(2009b):78-81, with the permission from Elsevier as the authors` right.

Several studies suggest the possibility that an interaction between glutamate and monoamine seems to exist in the prefrontal cortex (Gruss et al., 1999; Jedema and Moghaddam, 1996). In support of this interaction, microdialysis studies have suggested that DA release in the prefrontal cortex induced by stress was, in part, a consequence of an increased glutamatergic neurotransmission (Del Arco et al., 1999; Jedema and Moghaddam, 1993; Takahata and Maghaddam, 1998). However, other studies did not support this claim, because it has been shown that stress did not increase extracellular concentrations of glutamate in the prefrontal cortex (Del Arco and Mora, 2001; Timmerman et al., 1999). Thus, the release of monoamine during stress in the prefrontal cortex is still controversial. The present results indicated that L-Pro might be involved in the release of monoamines during stress in the prefrontal cortex mediated by the NMDA receptor. Indeed, there is a long history of evidence suggesting that L-Pro may be a neuronal modulator or transmitter in the central nervous system (Fremeau et al., 1992; Gogos et al., 1999; Renick et al., 1999; Snyder et al., 1973; Yoneda and Roberts, 1982). It is known that L-Pro containing neurons and transporters are localized in several brain areas (Fremeau et al., 1992; Renick et al., 1999; Takemoto and Semba, 2006). However, the effect of stress on extracellular L-Pro is still obscure. Further study is necessary to verify the hypothesis.

Acknowledgments

This work was supported by a Grant-in-Aid for Scientific Research from Japan Society for the Promotion of Science (Nos. 13460118, 14206033, 16380191, 17208023, 18208023 and 21380165) and the SKYLARK Food Science Institute.

References

Abercrombie, E.D., Keefe, K.A., Difrischia, D.S. and Zigmond, M.J., Differential effect of stress on in vivo dopamine release in striatum, nucleus accumbens, and medial frontal cortex, *J. Neurochem*., 52(1989):1655-1658.

Arco, A.D. and Mora, F., Dopamine release in the prefrontal cortex during stress is reduced by the local activation of glutamate receptors, *Brain Res. Bull.*, 56(2001): 125-130.

Asechi, M., Tomonaga, S., Tachibana, T., Han, L., Hayamizu, K., Denbow, D.M. and Furuse, M., Intracerebroventricular injection of L-serine analogs and derivatives induces sedative and hypnotic effects under an acute stressful condition in neonatal chicks, *Behav. Brain Res.*, 170(2006):71-77.

Baquet, A., Lavoinne, A. and Hue, L., Comparison of the effects of various amino acids on glycogen synthesis, lipogenesis and ketogenesis in isolated rat hepatocytes, *J. Biochem.*, 273(1991):57-62.

Bhatnagar, S., Costall, B. and Smythe, J.W., Hippocampal cholinergic blockade enhances hypothalamic-pituitary-adrenal responses to stress, *Brain Res.*, 766(1997):244-248.

Boehning, D. and Snyder, S.H., Novel neural modulators, *Annu. Rev. Neurosci.*, 26(2003):105-131.

Cohen, S.M. and Nadler, J.V., Proline-induced potentiation of glutamate transmission, *Brain Res.*, 761 (1997):271-282.

David, M., Brian, A. and Victor, N., NMDA receptor-mediated depolarizing action of proline on CA1 pyramidal cells, *Eur. J. Pharmacol.*, 219(1992):59-66.

Davis, J.L., Masuoka, D.T., Gerbrandt, L.K. and Cherkin, A., Autoradiographic distribution of L-proline in chicks after intracerebral injection, *Physiol. Behav.*, 22(1979):693-695.

Degroot, A. and Parent, M.B., Infusion of physostigmine into the hippocampus or the entorhinal cortex attenuate avoidance retention deficits produced by intra-septal infusions of the GABA agonist muscimol, *Brain Res.*, 920(2001):10-18.

Degroot, A., Kashluba, S. and Treit, D., Septal GABAergic and hippocampal cholinergic systems modulate anxiety in the plus-maze and shock-probe tests, *Pharmacol. Biochem. Behav.*, 69(2001): 391-399.

Del Arco, A., Gonzalez-Mora, J.L., Armas, V.R. and Mora, F., Amphetamine increases extracellular concentrations of glutamate in striatum of the awake rat, *Neuropharmacology*, 38(1999):943-954.

Del Arco, A. and Mora, F., Dopamine release in the prefrontal cortex during stress is reduced by the local activation of glutamate receptors, *Brain Res. Bull.*, 56(2001): 125-130.

Delwing, D., Chiarani, F., Delwing, D., Bavaresco, C.S., Wannmacher, C.M., Wajner, M. and Wyse, A.T., Proline reduces acetylcholinesterase activity in cerebral cortex of rats, *Metab. Brain Dis.*, 18(2003): 79-86.

Doherty, M.D. and Gratton, A., Effects of medial prefrontal cortical injections of GABA receptor agonists and antagonists on the local and nucleus accumbens dopamine responses to stress, *Synapse*, 32(1999):288-300.

Farah, J.M. Jr, Rao, T.S., Mick, S.J., Coyne, K.E. and Iyengar, S., N-methyl-D-aspartate treatment increases circulating adrenocorticotropin and luteinizing hormone in the rat, *Endocrinology*, 128(1991):1875-1880.

Feltenstein, M.W., Lambdin, L.C., Ganzera, M., Ranjith, H., Dharmaratne, W. and Nanayakkara, N.P., Anxiolytic properties of Piper methysticum extract samples and fractions in the chick social-separation-stress procedure, *Phytother. Res.*, 17(2003): 210-216.

Fremeau, R.T. Jr, Caron, M.G. and Blakely, R.D., Molecular cloning and expression of a high affinity L-proline transporter expressed in putative glutamatergic pathways of rat brain, *Neuron*, 8(1992):915-926.

Gogos, J.A., Sautha, M., Takacs, Z., Beck, K.D., Luine, V., Lucas, L.R., Nadler, J.V. and Karayiorgou, M., The gene encoding proline dehydrogenase modulates sensorimotor gating in mice, *Nat. Genet.*, 21(1999):434-439.

Gruss, M. and Braun, K., Distinct activation of monoaminergic pathways in chick brain in relation to auditory imprinting and stressful situations: a microdialysis study, *Neuroscience*, 76(1996):891-899.

Gruss, M., Bredenkotter, M. and Braun, K., N-methyl-D-aspartate receptor-mediated modulation of monoaminergic metabolites and amino acids in the chick forebrain: an in vivo microdialysis and electrophysiology study, *J. Neurobiol.*, 40(1999): 116-135.

Halpain, S., Wieczorek, C.M. and Rainbow, T.C., Localization of L-glutamate receptors in rat brain by quantitative autoradiography, *J. Neurosci.*, 4(1984):2247-2258.

Hamasu, K., Haraguchi, T., Kabuki, Y., Adachi, N., Tomonaga, S., Sato, H., Denbow, D.M. and Furuse, M., L-Proline is a sedative regulator of acute stress in the brain of neonatal chicks, *Amino Acids*, 37 (2009a):377-382.

Hamasu, K., Kabuki, Y., Tomonaga, S., Denbow, D.M. and Furuse, M., Changes in brain monoamine metabolism of neonatal chicks under two different acute stress conditions, *Br. Poult. Sci.*, 53 (2012):145-149.

Hamasu, K., Shigemi, K., Kabuki, Y., Tomonaga, S., Denbow, D.M. and Furuse, M., Central L-proline attenuates stress-induced dopamine and serotonin metabolism in the chick forebrain, *Neurosci. Lett.*, 460(2009b):78-81.

Hamasu, K., Shigemi, K., Tsuneyoshi, Y., Sato, H., Denbow, D.M. and Furuse, M., Cholinergic neurotransmission is not involved in sedation induced by L-proline in neonatal chicks. *J. Anim. Vet. Adv.*, 8(2009c):1207-1211.

Hamasu, K., Shigemi, K., Tsuneyoshi, Y., Yamane, H., Sato, H., Denbow, D.M. and Furuse, M., Intracerebroventricular injection of L-proline and D-proline induces sedative and hypnotic effects by different mechanisms under an acute stressful condition in chicks, *Amino Acids*, 38(2010):57-64.

Haraguchi, T., Tomonaga, S., Kurauchi, I., Hamasu, K., Sato, H., Denbow, D.M. and Furuse, M., Intracerebroventricular injection of L-proline modifies food intake in neonatal chicks, *J. Anim. Vet. Adv.*, 6(2007):1255-1257.

Henzi, V., Reichling, D.B., Helm, S.W. and MacDermott, A.B., L-Proline activates glutamate and glycine receptors in cultured rat dorsal horn neurons, *Mol. Pharmacol.*, 41(1992):793-801.

Hess, C. and Blozovski, D., Hippocampal muscarinic cholinergic mediation of spontaneous alternation and fear in the developing rat, *Behav. Brain Res.,* 24(1987): 203-214.

Hu, C.A., Phang, J.M. and Valle, D., Proline metabolism in health and disease, *Amino Acids*, 35(2008):651-652.

Jedema, H.P. and Moghaddam, B., Glutamatergic control of dopamine release during stress in the rat prefrontal cortex, *J. Neurochem.*, 63(1993):785-788.

Jedema, H.P. and Moghaddam, B., Characterization of excitatory amino acid modulation of dopamine release in the prefrontal cortex of conscious rats, *J. Neurochem.*, 66(1996):1448-1453.

Jezová, D., Tokarev, D. and Rusnák, M., Endogenous excitatory amino acids are involved in stress-induced adrenocorticotropin and catecholamine release, *Neuroendocrinology*, 62(1995):326-332.

Joanny, P., Steinberg, J., Oliver, C. and Grino, M., Glutamate and N-methyl-D-aspartate stimulate rat hypothalamic corticotropin-releasing factor secretion in vitro, *J. Neuroendocrinol.*, 9(1997):93-97.

Koutoku, T., Takahashi, H., Tomonaga, S., Oikawa, D., Saito, S., Tachibana, T., Han, L., Hayamizu, K., Denbow, D.M. and Furuse, M., Central administration of phosphatidylserine attenuates isolation stress induced behavior in chicks, *Neurochem. Int.*, 47(2005):183-189.

Kurauchi, I, Asechi, M., Tachibana, T., Han, L., Hayamizu, K., Denbow, D.M. and Furuse, M., Intracerebroventricular injection of L-alanine induces a sedative effect under an acute stressful condition in neonatal chicks, *J. Poult. Sci.*, 43(2006):384-387.

Kurata, K., Shigemi, K., Tomonaga, S., Aoki, M., Morishita, K., Denbow, D.M. and Furuse, M., L-Ornithine attenuates corticotropin-releasing factor-induced stress responses acting at GABAA receptors in neonatal chicks, *Neuroscience*, 172(2011):226-231.

Lindstrom, P. and Ohlsson, L., Effect of N-methyl-D, L-aspartate on isolated rat somatotrophs, *Endocrinology*, 131(1992):1903-1907.

Mahesh, V.B., Zamorano, P., Sevilla, L.D., Lewis, D. and Brann, D.V., Characterization of ionotropic glutamate receptors in rat hypothalamus, pituitary and immortalized gonadotropin-releasing hormone (GnRH) neurons (GT1-7 cells), *Neuroendocrinology*, 69(1999):397-407.

Metzger, M., Jiang, S. and Braun, K., A quantitative immuno-electron microscopic study of dopamine terminals in forebrain regions of the domestic chick involved in filial imprinting, *Neuroscience*, 111(2002):611-623.

Metzger, M., Jiang, S., Wang, J. and Braun, K., Organisation of the dopaminergic innervation of forebrain areas relevant to learning: A combined immuno-histochemical/retrograde tracing study in the domestic chick, *J. Comp. Neurol.*, 376(1996):1-27.

Muller, S.C. and Scheich, H., Social stress increases [^{14}C]2-deoxyglucose incorporation in three rostral forebrain areas of the young chick, *Behav. Brain Res.*, 19(1986):93-98.

Ortiz, J.G., Cordero, M.L. and Rosado, A., Proline-glutamate interactions in the CNS, *Prog. Neuropsychopharmacol. Biol. Psychiatry*, 21(1996):141-152.

Panksepp, J., Meeker, R. and Bean, N.J., The neurochemical control of crying. *Pharmacol. Biochem. Behav.*, 12(1980a): 437-443.

Panksepp, J., Bean, N.J., Bishop, P., Vilberg, T.and Sahley, T.L., Opioid blockade and social comfort in chicks, *Pharmacol. Biochem. Behav.*, 13(1980b):673-683.

Renick, S.E., Kleven, D.T., Chan, J., Stenius, K., Milner, T.A., Pickel, V.M. and Fremeau, R.T. Jr, The mammalian brain high-affinity L-proline transporter is enriched preferentially in synaptic vesicles in a subpopulation of excitatory nerve terminals in rat forebrain, *J. Neurosci.*, 19(1999): 21-33.

Sahley, T.L., Panksepp, J. and Zolovick, A.J., Cholinergic modulation of separation distress in the domestic chick, *Eur. J. Pharmacol.*, 72(1981):261-264.

Santiago, M., Machado, A. and Cano, J., Regulation of the prefrontal cortical dopamine release by GABAa and GABAb receptor agonists and antagonists, *Brain Res.*, 630(1993):28-31.

Smythe, J.W., Bhatnagar, S., Murphy, D., Timothy, C. and Costall, B., The effects of intrahippocampal scopolamine infusion on anxiety in rats as measured by the black-white box test, *Brain Res. Bull.*, 45(1998): 89-93.

Snyder, S.H., Young, A.B., Bennett, J.P. and Mulder, A.H., Synaptic biochemistry of amino acids, *Fed. Proc.*, 32(1973):2039-2047.

Suenaga, R., Tomonaga, S., Yamane, H., Kurauchi, I., Tsuneyoshi, Y., Sato, H., Denbow, D.M. and Furuse, M., Intracerebroventricular injection of L-arginine induces sedative and hypnotic effects under an acute stress in neonatal chicks, *Amino Acids*, 35(2008a):139-146.

Suenaga, R., Yamane, H., Tomonaga, S., Asechi, M., Adachi, N., Tsuneyoshi, Y., Kurauchi, I., Sato, H., Denbow, D.M. and Furuse, M., Central L-arginine reduced stress responses are mediated by L-ornithine in neonatal chicks, *Amino Acids*, 35(2008b):107-113.

Sugden, M.C., Watts, D.I., West, P.S. and Palmer, T.N., Proline and hepatic lipogenesis, *Biochim. Biophys. Acta*, 798(1984):368-373.

Takagi, T., Ando, R., Ohgushi, A., Yamashita, T., Dobashi, E., Hussain-Yusuf, H., Onodera, R., Bungo, T., Sato, H. and Furuse, M., Intracerebroventricular injection of pipecolic acid inhibits food intake and induces sleeping-like behaviors in the neonatal chick, *Neurosci. Lett.*, 310(2001):97-100.

Takagi, T., Bungo, T., Tachibana, T., Saito, E.-S., Saito, S., Yamasaki, I., Tomonaga, S., Denbow, D.M. and Furuse, M., Intracerebroventricular administration of GABA-A and GABA-B receptor antagonists attenuate feeding and sleep-like behavior induced by L-pipecolic acid in the neonatal chick, *J. Neurosci. Res.*, 73(2003a):270-275.

Takagi, T., Tachibana, T., Saito, E.-S., Tomonaga, S., Saito, S., Bungo, T., Denbow, D.M. and Furuse, M., Central pipecolic acid increases food intake under ad libitum feeding conditions in the neonatal chick, *Neurosci. Lett.*, 347(2003b):93-96.

Takahata, R. and Moghaddam, B., Glutamatergic regulation of basal and stimulus-activated dopamine release in the prefrontal cortex, *J. Neurochem.*, 71(1998):1443-1449.

Takemoto, Y., Depressor responses to L-proline microinjected into the rat ventrolateral medulla are mediated by ionotropic excitatory amino acid receptors, *Auton. Neurosci.*, 120(2005):108-112.

Takemoto, Y. and Semba, R., Immunohistochemical evidence for the localization of neurons containing the putative transmitter L-proline in rat brain, *Brain Res.*, 1073-1074(2006):311-315.

Timmerman, W., Cisci, G., Nap, A., De Vries, J.B. and Westerink, B.H., Effects of handling on extracellular levels of glutamate and other amino acids in various areas of the brain measured by microdialysis, *Brain Res.*, 833 (1999) 150-160.

Tomonaga, S., Denbow, D.M. and Furuse, M. Central functions of L-arginine and its metabolites for stress behavior. In: *Arginine Amino Acid* (Edited by Nathan L. Jacobs), pp. 163-189. NOVA Science Publishers Inc., Hauppauge NY, USA. (2011)

Tomonaga, S., Tachibana, T., Takagi, T., Saito, E.-S., Zhang, R., Denbow, D.M. and Furuse, M., Effect of central administration of carnosine and its constituents on behaviors in chicks, *Brain Res. Bull.*, 63(2004):75-82.

Van Luijtelaar, E.L.J.M., van der Grinten, C.P.M., Blokhuis, H.J. and Coenen, A.M.L., Sleep in the domestic hen (*Gallus domesticus*), *Physiol. Behav.*, 41(1987): 409-414.

Yamane, H., Tsuneyoshi, Y., Denbow, D.M. and Furuse, M., *N*-Methyl-*D*-aspartate and α-amino-3-hydroxy-5-methyl-4-isoxazolepropionate receptors involved in the induction of sedative effects under an acute stress in neonatal chicks. *Amino Acids*, 37(2009):733-739. *Erratum*, 37(2009):767.

Yoneda, S and Roberts, E., A new synaptosomal biosynthetic pathway of proline from ornithine and its negative feedback inhibition by proline, *Brain Res.*, 239 (1982): 479-488.

In: Proline
Editor: Bouzid Nedjimi

ISBN: 978-1-62257-739-2

Chapter VII

Tumor Suppressor Activities of Proline Oxidase

Steve A. Maxwell*
Department of Molecular & Cellular Medicine,
College of Medicine,College Station, TX, US

Abstract

Proline oxidase (POX) is a p53-regulated redox gene that mediates tumor suppression by inducing cell cycle arrest and proline-dependent apoptosis. A degenerate p53 consensus binding site in the POX promoter allows the gene to respond to p53. POX functions as a mitochondrial tumor suppressor by inducing intrinsic and extrinsic apoptosis, mediating a G2 cell cycle arrest, and reducing hypoxia-inducible factor (HIF) signaling. Consistent with its role as a tumor suppressor, POX expression levels are frequently much lower in renal, colorectal, pancreatic, liver, and stomach tumor tissues than in their normal tissue counterparts. The loss of POX is not due to genetic or epigenetic mechanisms but instead occurs through upregulation of the mir-23b microRNA, which suppresses translation of POX mRNA by binding to its 3' untranslated region. P53-induced POX generates reactive oxygen species (ROS) through oxidation of proline. Pyrroline-5-carboxylate, the product of proline oxidation, is recycled back to proline with

* Department of Molecular & Cellular Medicine, Rm. 252 College of Medicine, College Station, TX 77843-1114, smaxwell@medicine.tamhsc.edu

redox transfers or converted to glutamate and a-ketoglutarate; the latter enhances the prolyl hydroxylation of HIF and its proteasomal degradation. POX mediates the activation of the NFAT transcription factor by p53 through activation of the calcium/calmodulin-dependent phosphatase, calcineurin. POX-induced ROS mobilizes calcium from intracellular stores to activate calcineurin, which then activates the NFAT transcription factor to modulate gene expression and apoptosis. The initiation of calcineurin-regulated transcription factor pathways may affect gene expression events important in not only apoptosis but other p53-regulated physiological processes. POX also mediates p53-independent signaling pathways. Peroxisome proliferator-activated receptor ligands mediate apoptosis in human lung cancers by inducing POX. Upregulation of POX expression dramatically decreases phosphorylation of MEK and ERK, which is partially reversed by expression of manganese superoxide dismutase. Overexpression of a constitutively active form of MEK suppressed POX-induced apoptosis, suggesting the involvement of MEK/ERK signaling and further confirming the role of ROS/superoxides in POX-induced apoptosis. Etoposide, a conventional anticancer drug, upregulates p53, POX, NFAT, and ROS, and induces apoptosis, in responsive tumor cells. The involvement of POX in both p53-dependent and -independent tumor suppressor pathways makes it an attractive strategic target for cancer therapy in a variety of human cancers.

The Proline Cycle

Proline metabolism has progressively become realized as playing a major role in human health and disease over the past 40 years (1-8). Proline originates from its direct precursor, Δ^1-pyrroline-5-carboxylate (Δ^1P5C), which is derived from the amino acid L-glutamate (1, 2, 5). Proline is an abundant amino acid, which, together with hydroxyproline, comprises more than 25% of collagen residues, the most abundant protein in the human body (3). The proline- Δ^1P5C cycle mediates a critical role in the regulation of gene expression, apoptosis, cell growth, purine biosynthesis, and cellular redox state (5-10).

Proline has a unique structure that prevents it from being a substrate for enzymes metabolizing most amino acids. The amino acid has evolved with its own metabolizing system (*Figure 1*). Proline oxidase (POX), also known as proline dehydrogenase (PRODH), is a mitochondrial inner-membrane enzyme involved in the metabolism of proline to pyrroline-5-carboxylate (Δ^1P5C) (5, 11). Δ^1P5C is reduced to proline by P5C reductase in the cytoplasm and the reverse reaction is performed by POX, which is located in the inner mitochondrial membrane. These reactions, when coupled with the conversion of Δ^1P5C to proline by P5C reductase, mediate the proline cycle to shuttle redox equivalents between mitochondria and the cytosol (5, 10, 12-14). The pair of electrons donated by proline can be used either for direct reduction of oxygen to form superoxide or is transferred into the electron transport chain for ATP production. Δ^1P5C provides a direct carbon bridge connecting proline metabolism with the tricarboxylic cycle through glutamate and α-ketoglutarate (5). Changes in the cycling of proline through POX can alter the redox balance via the production of reactive oxygen species, critical for regulation of cell growth and apoptosis (12, 15-19). POX mediates mitochondria-induced apoptosis with the release of cytochrome c, activation of caspase-9, followed by DNA fragmentation, chromatin condensation, and cell shrinkage (12, 15-17, 19-24).

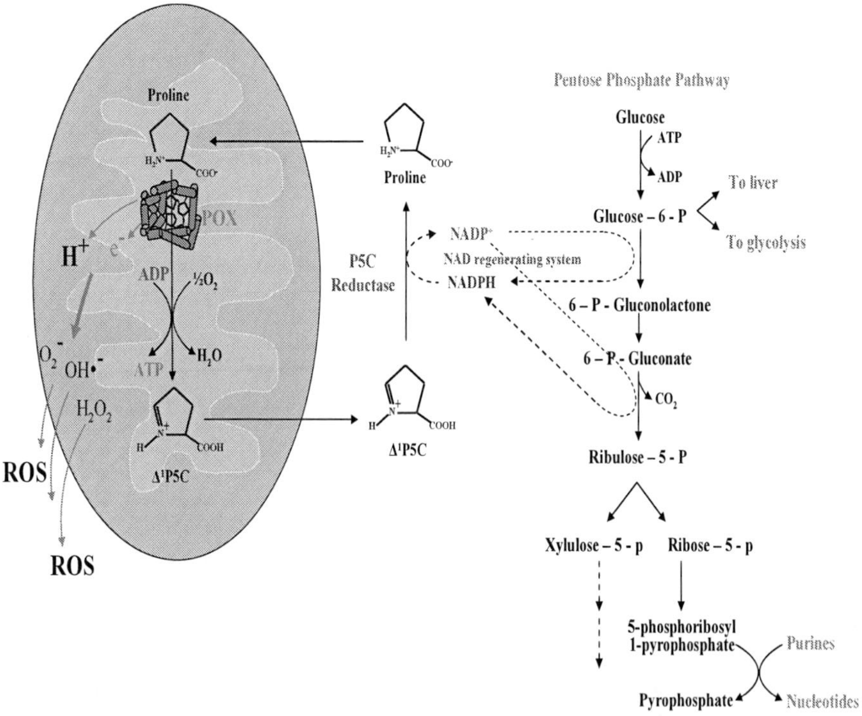

Figure 1. The proline cycle. Proline oxidase converts proline to Δ^1P5C coupled to the production of ATP. Δ^1P5C is shuttled to the cytoplasm and reduced to proline by P5C reductase; this reduction is coupled to the oxidation of NAD which drives the pentose phosphate pathway and the production of purines. POX also donates protons and electrons to the mitochondrial respiratory chain that eventually will lead to the production of free radicals (ROS). [201, 202].

Upregulation of POX enables cells to undergo an L-proline-dependent apoptotic response (15). In the presence of proline, high POX activity was sufficient to induce mitochondria-mediated apoptosis (15). These apoptotic effects can be blocked by the forced expression of the CuZn-form of superoxide dismutase (SOD2) but not the Mn superoxide dismutase form (SOD1) (16).

POX is located in a strategic position in the middle of glutamate pathway, which is the basic molecule for production of ribonucleotides (5, 8, 25). Additionally, the mitochondrial-cytoplasmic proline-Δ^1P5C shuttle participates in the NADPH regenerating system, which transfers the electrons that it has gained from the oxidation of glucose to molecular oxygen forming water, thereby releasing chemical energy that is used to make ATP (14, 26, 27). In normal tissue, Δ^1P5C and proline form a catalytic cycle where they mediate redox transfers between mitochondria and cytosol regulating several pathways (5, 16, 28). The actions of POX and Δ^1P5C reductase enhance the production of ribose and phosphoribosylpyrophosphate for ribonucleotides synthesis (5, 25, 29), regulate hypoxia-induced gene expression (20, 30), and modulate both extrinsic and intrinsic programmed cell death in cells undergoing p53-mediated apoptosis via ROS production (9, 12, 15, 17, 18, 20, 21, 23, 24, 31). Proline metabolized by POX can be used as a stress substrate and sensor for survival or apoptosis (6, 10, 32, 33). The process of activation of matrix metalloproteinases and prolidase, which degrade the collagen contained in extracellular matrix to furnish proline for POX, has been designated the term, "ecophagy" (6, 28).

Proline Oxidase (POX/PRODH) Gene Structure

The human PRODH1 (GeneID: 5625) structural gene is localized at 17.3 Mb on chromosome 22q11.21, which is comprised of 15 exons spanning 23.77 kb and encodes a 600-amino acid POX protein (34). The POX gene is evolutionarily conserved with a high degree of homology existing among evolutionarily-diverse species including drosophila, zebrafish, mouse, rat, and human. A PRODH1 pseudogene (ΨPOX), located 1.4 Mb telomeric on 22q at 18.7 Mb, has >95% sequence identity with POX but has an internal deletion that removes a 13.1-kb segment containing exons 2 through the 5′ half of exon 7, along with the intervening introns (35, 36). ΨPOX has accumulated several missense mutations that, in some instances, have been transferred to POX, apparently by gene conversion (35).

Missense mutations in the PRODH1 gene are associated with multiple disease states, including type I hyperprolinemia (HPI), non-specified hyperprolinemia, velocardiofacial syndrome/DiGeorge syndrome (VCFS/DGS), CATCH 22 syndrome, and schizophrenia (37, 38). At least 16 POX missense mutations have been identified in patients with hyperprolinemia, schizophrenia, and control subjects (35, 39). The functional consequences of these missense mutations have been deduced by evolutionary conservation of the altered residue. Lately, those missense mutations have been tested directly *in vitro* (40). Four alleles result in mild, six in moderate, and five in severe reduction in POX activity, whereas one increases POX activity. There is some evidence that severe hyperprolinemia occurs in individuals with large deletions and/or POX missense mutations, whereas the less severe cases of hyperprolinemia are associated with POX alleles exhibiting a milder reduction in activity. With respect to cancer, mutations in POX/PRODH1 have not been observed. Instead, loss of POX in renal cancers can occur by dysregulation of a microRNA (30).

Regulation of the POX/PRODH Gene

Practically all cell types, with the exception of red blood cells, express POX (5, 41, 42). In pigs, POX activity is highest in the small intestine, followed by liver, kidney, and placenta (41, 43). POX is expressed ubiquitously in the human, with the highest expression in the brain, spinal cord, heart, skeletal muscle, liver, kidney, and lung. In adult rats, POX activity is highest in the liver and kidney with moderate expression in the brain and heart. No POX activity is detectable in the lung, skeletal muscle, spleen, or small intestine (44). During development, the activity of POX changes, undergoing increases in the liver and kidney as rats mature from fetal to adult life (45). Under conditions of nutrient stress, POX/PRODH is upregulated by a mechanism involving the mTOR-signaling system. Dysfunction of POX can result in abnormally high serum proline levels (46). Disease states such as cancer result from loss or deficiency in POX activity, thus implicating it as a tumor suppressor.

POX was identified as a p53-induced gene by serial analysis of gene expression (SAGE) (18). Maxwell and Davis (22) also identified POX as a p53-regulated gene and were the first to report that Δ^1P5C could mediate apoptosis, thus implicating POX as a potential mediator of p53-dependent apoptosis via ROS. P53 is a central tumor suppressor protein that regulates the processes of cell cycling, angiogenesis, differentiation, bioenergetics, and apoptosis (47-49). In the study by Polyak et al. (18), p53 overexpression induced 14 genes, termed PIGs. POX was designated as the PIG6 gene. Two other proline metabolic enzymes, Δ^1P5C dehydrogenase and Δ^1P5C synthetase, have been shown to be upregulated by p53 (50).

A p53-binding site is positioned at –1161 to –1188 upstream of the POX gene, implicating the POX gene as a direct target in p53-dependent generation of ROS and induction of apoptosis (51). The p53-binding site in the POX promoter was identified by chromatin-immunoprecipitation (ChIP) assays using p53 monoclonal antibodies. A sequence analysis of the POX gene (PRODH; GenBank NM_016335.2) and its 5' flanking sequences revealed a potential p53 binding site, GGGCTTGTCTTCGTGTGACTTCTGTCT, beginning 1,161 base pairs upstream of the transcriptional start site. A 711-bp PRODH1 upstream fragment containing the candidate p53-binding site exhibited reporter gene activity that was induced by p53. In contrast, the same DNA region lacking the candidate p53 binding site did not show significant p53-response activity. Electrophoretic mobility shift assay (EMSA) in the presence of p53 antibodies confirmed that p53 could directly bind to the *PRODH1* upstream sequence containing the candidate p53-binding site.

Transcription factors regulating the PRODH promoter have been identified by transfection of a *PRODH* promoter-luciferase reporter construct into several colorectal cancer cell lines (17). Transcription factors were co-transfected with the *PRODH* promoter-luciferase reporter to screen for activators of the *PRODH* promoter. The peroxisomal proliferator-activated receptor gamma (PPARγ) was identified as the most potent activator of the PRODH promoter. Modest activation of the *PRODH1* promoter was observed with c-Jun, c-Fos, and P-65 of NFκB. The PRODH promoter was activated more than 10-fold by PPARγ ligands (thiazolidinedione, TZD), in a variety of different colorectal cancer cells. EMSA and ChiP assays confirmed that PPARγand its ligands directly upregulate the expression of the *PRODH* gene through transactivation of its promoter. The integration of signaling by the PPARγ complex assembly to regulate *PRODH* expression may be more complex under physiological conditions, since it is known that its interaction with co-factor retinoid-X receptors (RXR) is required for PPARγ function (52).

POX can activate protective autophagy critical in the cellular response to the noxious effects of oxidized low density lipoproteins (53). OxLDLs exhibited cytotoxicity and activated both apoptosis and autophagy in both colon (HT29) and prostate (PC3) carcinoma cells. OxLDLs interact with PPARγ and were found to upregulate proline oxidase (POX) through this nuclear receptor, particularly through the 7-ketocholesterol ligand. Knock-down of POX decreased OxLDLassociated ROS generation and decreased autophagy as measured via beclin-1 protein level and conversion of light-chain 3 protein (LC3)-I into LC3-II. Upregulation of POX was sufficient to activate autophagy, leading to the accumulation of autophagosomes. Beclin-1 gene expression was directly dependent on the generation of POX-dependent superoxide. Although POX was initially found to mediate the apoptotic process downstream of p53 (18), HT29 expresses a mutant p53 and PC3 has no p53, thus implicating the POX-dependent regulation of autophagy as a p53-independent process (53).

The loss of POX expression in cancer can be mediated by microRNAs (miRNAs). One specific type of miRNA, termed miR-23b, has been shown to repress POX expression. Knockdown of miR-23b resulted in the upregulation of POX, resulting in ROS-induced apoptosis along with decreased HIF-1α signaling in renal cancer cells (30).

The metabolic and bioenergetic pathways, such as glycolysis and oxidative phosphorylation, respectively, have critical roles in cancer (54, 55). Pathways that maintain bioenergetics involved with survival after starvation also play important roles (56). One such pathway involves release of proline from collagen in the extracellular matrix, which provides substrates for ATP generation (6, 10, 29). Since up to 25% of the residues in collagen are proline and hydroxyproline, its degradation by metalloproteinases (MMPs) and prolidase during inflammation and tumorigenesis releases large amounts of proline (1, 2, 6, 10, 28, 33). Tumorigenesis, genotoxic stress, inflammation, and nutrient stress can upregulate MMPs (57-60), which leads to upregulation of POX. The proline in collagen provides a microenvironmental stress resource for POX to regulate bioenergetics and survival (6, 9). HIF signaling is also affected, which can regulate angiogenesis and tumor progression (30, 61).

POX-Regulated Pathways

Oxidative Stress

Upregulation of POX can generate increases in proline-dependent ROS production (15, 16, 19, 20). ROS can mediate changes in gene expression by functioning as intracellular second messengers in signaling cascades involving Ca^{+2} (62). The induction of ROS by POX may very well mediate the influence that p53 has on calcium-signaling pathways that induce apoptosis. For instance, the induction of POX by p53 increases production of ROS, and ROS, in turn, can promote Ca^{+2} influx into the cytoplasm from intracellular stores such as the endoplasmic reticulum (63). Ca^{+2} mobilization activates calmodulin/calcineurin, which plays important roles as a multifunctional regulator of apoptosis (64, 65). The calcineurin phosphatase dephosphorylates the nuclear factor of activated T cells (NFAT) transcription factor complex, causing it to undergo translocation from the cytoplasm to the nucleus, where it regulates genes whose promoters contain NFAT binding sites such as Fas (66, 67).

The mechanisms regulating the production and targeting of ROS signals in apoptosis are not clear. The generation of ROS requires a functional mitochondrial respiratory chain in most ROS-dependent apoptotic death systems (68, 69). The functional linkage of POX at the inner mitochondrial membrane to cytochrome *c* in the electron transport chain (5, 9, 14, 25, 70) might be an important apoptotic control mechanism whereby POX could influence electron flow to support ROS production. Upregulation of POX expression by p53 would accelerate the proline redox cycle and thus result in increases in the amount of electrons delivered to the electron transport chain. The mechanism of POX-induced ROS generation might be leakage of excess electrons from the electron transport chain due to the increased leakage of acceptor cytochrome c from the mitochondria at the early stage of apoptosis. Indeed, increases in ROS production can lead to a process termed ROS-induced ROS release (RIRR) (71). RIRR is initiated by ROS acting to induce the opening of one of the requisite mitochondrial pore channels, which in turn produces a collapse of mitochondrial $\Delta\psi$. The collapse of the $\Delta\psi$ is followed by additional transient increases in ROS that are generated by the electron transfer chain. The release of a secondary ROS burst to the cytosol could potentially activate RIRR in neighboring mitochondria, which is then followed by the initiation of Ca^{+2} fluxes into the cytosol from intracellular storage compartments such as the endoplasmic reticulum and mitochondria. Increased cytoplasmic mobilization of Ca^{+2} might explain why calcineurin, a calcium-dependent protein phosphatase, is activated in response to upregulation of POX by ectopic means or chemotherapeutic agents (24).

Although POX-mediated, proline-dependent generation of superoxide is the result of electron leakage from the electron transport chain, studies from structural biology suggest that superoxide may be generated by an intrinsic activity of the enzyme (72). The bifunctional POX from prokaryotic species such as *Escherichia coli* exhibit the activities of proline oxidase and P5C dehydrogenase in a single protein. In contrast, the recombinant *Thermus thermophilus* POX is monofunctional and produces P5C in a manner similar to the enzyme in animal tissues. This monofunctional POX has the flavin adenine dinucleotide in a domain exposed to solvent oxygen. Moreover, an adjacent α-helix can shield the FAD and block its access to solvent oxygen. Under certain conditions, POX may be able to switch from an ATP-generating function to a superoxide-generating activity.

Extrinsic Death Receptor Pathway

An alternative apoptotic pathway known as the "death receptor" or "extrinsic" pathway involves ligands such as the tumor necrosis factor (TNF), TNF-related apoptosis-inducing ligand (TRAIL) and Fas ligand, which bind to their respective membrane receptors and recruit an adaptor molecule, the Fas-associated death domain (FADD) to activate caspase 8 and downstream caspases (73). Upregulation of POX in DLD-1 colon carcinoma cells induced expression of TRAIL, DR5, and cleavage of caspase-8 (21). A role for the extrinsic pathway in POX-mediated apoptosis was confirmed by the caspase-8 specific inhibitor, Z-IETD-FMK. These findings, along with the induction of TRAIL by POX, indicates that the extrinsic (death receptor) pathway is activated by POX, which may be mediated by NFAT transcription factors. Upregulation of POX activates NFAT, which then binds to and activates the promoter for TRAIL (21, 24, 74), resulting in activation of the extrinsic apoptotic pathway. POX thus induces potent apoptosis through both the intrinsic and extrinsic pathways and would be expected to induce apoptosis in a variety of different cell types.

Calcineurin/NFAT Pathway

Etoposide is an anti-cancer topoisomerase type II inhibitor that induces double-stranded breaks in DNA (75, 76). Inhibitors of topoisomerase II cause direct DNA damage by blocking DNA replication. Etoposide upregulates p53 and activates its DNA binding activity (77, 78). Induction of both p53 and POX, along with the activation of calcineurin, occurred in etoposide-treated ovarian and colon carcinoma cell lines undergoing apoptosis (23). A POX antisense and the calcineurin inhibitor FK506 inhibited the etoposide-mediated activation of calcineurin. Blocking calcineurin in the etoposide-treated cells reduced the incidence of apoptosis (23). Thus, the p53-dependent DNA damage response, in part, involves the induction of POX, which then generates ROS, stimulates release of Ca^{+2} from intracellular stores, leading to activation of calcineurin. Calcineurin can induce apoptosis by dephosphorylating and thus modulating the activity of different phosphoproteins that are involved in the apoptotic process such as Bcl-2 (79, 80) and Bad (81). Moreover, factors that modulate calcineurin activity can affect the expression of genes involved in apoptosis. For instance, Bcl-2 can mediate drug resistance and block apoptosis by binding and sequestering calcineurin, preventing the dephosphorylation of NFAT and preventing it from translocating to the nucleus (82). Without NFAT nuclear translocation, the FasL gene is not transcribed.

Since calcineurin is activated by POX and is capable of inducing cytochrome c release from the mitochondria into the cytoplasm, perhaps this is why cytochrome c release stimulated by p53 in renal and lung carcinoma cells was suppressed by the expression of a POX antisense (23). Superoxide dismutases, which are important antioxidant enzymes, were shown to inhibit POX-induced apoptosis and release of mitochondrial cytochrome c to the cytosol (16), further implicating the generation of superoxide radicals as playing a crucial role in POX-induced apoptosis. The proline oxidation pathway may be an alternative mechanism to the Bax/Bcl-2 pathway in mediating cytochrome c release by p53 in some cell types such as renal cells and in response to particular conditions of stress. Finally, it is of interest that the DNA binding of p53 to the HIV-1 long terminal repeats can be modulated by activated calcineurin [(83)]. Perhaps POX activates calcineurin, which then further activates p53 and/or alters the DNA binding specificity of p53 for gene targets.

Calcium can activate and inhibit gene transcription through members of the Ca^{+2}-binding EF-hand superfamily. Calmodulin and calcineurin are representative members of the EF-hand superfamily and can indirectly regulate transcription by influencing the phosphorylation state of transcription factors in response to increases in intracellular Ca^{+2} (84).

Based on the known effects of ROS on calcium levels in the cell, it has been proposed that POX can mediate changes in gene expression via ROS-induced mobilization of Ca^{+2}, which then activate calmodulin/calcineurin, leading to changes in the phosphorylation state and activities of transcription factors. The changes in transcription factor activity then lead to changes in gene expression that mediate, in part, p53-dependent apoptosis.

ROS generated by p53-induced POX have been suggested to be signaling molecules that activate the Ca^{+2}/calcineurin pathway and in turn activate NFAT as downstream events in p53-mediated apoptosis. Both p53 and POX activate NFAT through processes that are sensitive to calcium and ROS modifiers. Moreover, a POX antisense blocked p53-induced expression of POX and activation of NFAT, implicating POX as a direct downstream mediator of p53-induced activation of calcineurin.

MEK/ERK Pathway

The ability of the MAPK family to regulate apoptosis is dependent on the intracellular environment, which determines whether MAPK will induce or inhibit apoptosis. For example, depending on the cell type, p38 and JNK can either induce or inhibit apoptosis (85). An anti-apoptotic survival response is mediated by growth factors via the activation of the ERK pathway (85) and plays anti-apoptotic roles in the signaling of TNF, Fas, and TRAIL (85-88). MEK/ERK block apoptosis by inhibiting caspase-8 activation induced by ligand stimulation of death receptors (87, 89). Thus, no clear correlation exists between MAPK signaling and apoptosis.

POX is involved in regulation of the MEK/ERK pathway (21) most likely though ROS, since MAPK signaling is regulated by redox status. Phosphorylation of MEK and ERK was decreased by upregulation of POX, which was partially reversed by induction of manganese superoxide dismutase (MnSOD) (16). POX-induced apoptosis was inhibited by overexpression of a constitutively-active form of MEK (16). POX thus can mediate apoptosis through the inhibition of MEK/ERK signaling via ROS/superoxides (21).

Peroxisomal Proliferator Activated Receptor (PPAR) Pathway

The PPARγ pathway can exert a negative effect on cancer growth (90, 91). Activation of PPARγ by binding to ligands such as troglitazone results in reduced cell proliferation and induction of apoptosis (92). A reduced incidence of lung cancer has been detected in a population of patients with type 2 diabetes treated with PPARγ ligands (93). POX mediates the pro-apoptotic activities of PPARγ, as indicated by repression of PPARγ ligand-induced ROS production by anti-sense RNA knockdown of POX expression in colon carcinoma cells (17). The anticancer effect of PPARγ is dependent on a POX-induced p53-independent mechanism, which activates both mitochondrial (intrinsic) and death receptor pathways (17).

Hypoxia-Inducible Factor (HIF) Signaling

When in the presence of oxygen, cancer cells will switch glucose metabolism from respiration to lactic acid formation, which is known as the Warburg effect

(94). Activation of the hypoxia-inducible transcription factor (HIF-1α) leads to the reduced respiration rate and increased glucose uptake, which is associated with lactic acid production (95). Matrix metalloproteinases (MMPs) and prolidase catalyze collagen degradation to produce proline, which stimulates HIF-1α-signaling thereby influencing angiogenesis and tumor progression (61). POX represses HIF-1α-signaling by increasing α-ketoglutarate(α-KG), a crucial substrate for prolyl hydroxylase-catalyzed hydroxylation of HIF-1α and its degradation (20). P5C connects proline to the TCA cycle through glutamate and α-KG (5). α-KG dehydrogenase converts α-KG to succinyl-CoA, and is a target of ROS and oxidative stress (96). POX reduced HIF-1α and its downstream target, VEGF, under both normoxic and hypoxic conditions. α-KG dioxygenase controls the hydroxylation of proline and aspartate residues in the α-subunit of HIF-1α, which regulates its stability and transcriptional activity, allowing HIF-1α function as an oxygen sensor. HPLC analysis found increased levels of α-KG in POX-induced cells (20). The POX inhibition of HIF-1α was blocked by a cell-permeating α-KG analogue, providing additional evidence for a role of α-KG in POX-mediated regulation of HIF-1α signaling (20). Since the POX-mediated repression of HIF-1α was not inhibited by superoxide dismutase, it is most likely that α-KG, rather than superoxide, mediated POX regulation of HIF-1α signaling. The loss POX in tumor cells would eliminate the POX-mediated suppression of HIF-1α signaling, thus enhancing the switch to aerobic glycolysis, a characteristic of the Warburg effect (20).

Cyclooxygenase-2 (COX-2)

Dysregulation of COX-2-signaling is an important early step in colorectal tumorigenesis, making it an attractive target for cancer chemoprevention and treatment (97, 98). POX inhibited growth of colorectal carcinoma cells by repressing the production of prostaglandin E2 (PGE_2) and COX-2, which could be reversed by treatment with PGE_2 (12). Upregulation of POX led to decreased phosphorylation of EGFR and the addition of EGF partially reversed the POX-dependent downregulation of COX-2 expression. The increased amounts of COX-2 that are frequently observed in both premalignant and malignant tissues may be due to loss of POX expression. Growth factors, oncogenes, cytokines and tumor promoters may antagonize POX by promoting COX-2 transcription through protein kinase C- and Ras-mediated signaling. Moreover, a variety of transcription factors, including AP-1, NF-IL6, NF-κB, NFAT, and PEA3, activate COX-2 transcription depending on the cell type and inducing agent (99, 100). Wild type, but not mutant p53, can inhibit COX-2 transcription *in vitro* possibly through upregulation of POX. APC tumor suppressor gene status may also impact COX-2 expression (101). Thus, the balance between oncogenes and tumor suppressor genes, such as PRODH1, controls the expression of COX-2 in tumors.

Wnt/β -Catenin Pathway

Interactions among COX-2, β-catenin and the epidermal growth factor receptor (EGFR) are important for colorectal carcinogenesis (102-104). Wnt/β-catenin- signaling was repressed by POX, which led to reduced phosphorylation of glycogen synthase kinase-3beta (GSK-3β) and increased phosphorylation of β-catenin (12). The net result was decreased levels of β-catenin and lower β-catenin/TCF/LEF-mediated transcription. POX regulates the Wnt pathway through_COX-2/PGE_2 which transactivates the canonical APC/β-catenin/Wnt and EGFR signaling pathways through G protein-coupled receptors (103).

Pentose Phosphate Pathway

The pentose phosphate pathway is intimately connected to the proline cycle by NADPH/NADP+ through glucose-6-phosphate dehydrogenase (G6PDH) (25, 26, 105). Since the flux through G6PDH is controlled by the amount of NADP+ (106, 107), P5C reductase can be considered as a P5C-dependent NADPH dehydrogenase, which connects the proline cycle and the pentose phosphate pathway (108).

POX increases ATP, which is derived from NADPH produced by the pentose phosphate pathway (6, 9). In colorectal carcinoma cells, upregulation of POX activity had little effect on glycolysis but the pentose phosphate pathway was increased more than fivefold at all concentrations of glucose (28). Cells treated with dehydroepiandrosterone, a well-known inhibitor of G6PDH (109), the rate-limiting enzyme of the pentose phosphate pathway, markedly reduced the POX-dependent increase in cellular ATP (28). Thus, a significant amount of the increase in ATP is primarily connected to the generation of NADPH by the pentose phosphate pathway.

Cell Cycle Control

Tumor suppressor proteins mediate anti-cancer activity through either induction of apoptosis or blockage of the cell cycle, or both. Consistent with its role as a tumor suppressor, upregulation of POX induced a G2 cell cycle arrest (20). Three days after upregulation of POX, the amount of cells in sub-G_1/G_0 phase increased very little (from 2% to 4–6%). The most significant changes were in the S phase population, which decreased from 23% to 8%. The G_2 phase population increased from 18% to 39%, which indicated a G_2 cell cycle arrest induced by POX. Changes in the phosphorylation state of CDC2 appeared responsible for the POX-induced G2 cell cycle arrest. CDC2 is a cyclin-dependent kinase that promotes cells to proceed into mitosis. DNA damage targets CDC2 to cause a G2 arrest (110). Although total CDC2 did not change in POX-induced cells, the phosphorylation at tyrosine 15 of CDC2 increased, whereas phosphorylation at threonine 161 decreased, indicating an inactive status for CDC2 (20). CDC25C is the phosphatase that removes the inhibitory phosphates from CDC2 and activates cyclinB-CDC2 (110). CDC25C was found to be down-regulated in POX-induced cells thus implicating it as a POX target leading to inactivation of CDC2 (20).

Gene expression profiling by cDNA microarray identified most members of the GADD (growth arrest and DNA damage inducible gene) family to be upregulated in POX-induced cells (20). Of this family, GADD45α, GADDβ, GADDγ, and GADD34 were upregulated more than 3-fold. GADD45α is a downstream gene target of p53 and induces G2 arrest and, in some cases, apoptosis (111). Thus, POX most likely mediates G2 cell cycle arrest through CDC2 and GADD.

Loss of POX in Human Tumors

The functional loss of POX may promote resistance of tumor cells to apoptosis, thus driving tumor progression. A number of observations implicate POX as a tumor suppressor. First, POX participates in apoptosis induced by p53 in a variety of cancer cell types (12, 15-18, 24). Second, POX upregulation inhibits growth of cultured tumor cells and suppresses tumor formation in a xenograft model (12, 20). Third, POX expression is absent or reduced in a variety of human tumor tissues, including kidney, colon, stomach, liver and pancreas, as compared with their normal tissue counterparts (12, 20, 23). However, no genetic or epigenetic variation of the *PRODH1* gene and its promoter was observed in human tumor panels (30).

Maxwell and Rivera *et al.* (23) proposed that the reduced expression of POX mRNA in clear cell renal cancer was due to mutated p53. However, p53 mutation is an infrequent event in clear cell renal cell carcinoma (112, 113), which makes up the majority of kidney cancer cases. Furthermore, POX expression was reduced in both p53-mutant (786-0 and TK10) and p53 wild-type cell lines (UO31). Thus, the reduction of POX is likely due to some factor other than p53 status, since renal tumor cells had a much lower POX protein expression than normal renal cells even in the presence of equal expression of mRNA. In light of this, a microRNA designated as mirR23b, has been shown to regulate POX expression. Knockdown of miR-23b not only increased apoptosis by upregulating POX and superoxides, but also decreased HIF-1α signaling in renal cancer cells (30). Thus, miR-23b is an attractive therapeutic target in renal cell carcinoma.

Potential of POX as a Therapeutic Target in Cancer

Proline metabolism affects multiple signaling pathways that can influence both apoptosis and tumor progression. The loss of the tumor suppressive functions of POX decreases POX-mediated apoptosis, removes the POX-mediated suppression of HIF signaling, and promotes the conversion to aerobic glycolysis, one of the features of the Warburg effect (Figure 2). The multiple tumor suppressor properties exhibited make POX an attractive therapeutic target to control metabolism that is altered leading to the Warburg effect in tumor cells.

Moreover, proline stored in collagen serves as a microenvironmental stress sensor, leading to either survival or apoptosis. The extracellular matrix and tumor microenvironment are considered to be targets for cancer chemoprevention (114). Proline primarily derived from extracellular matrix after the digestion of collagen by MMPs and prolidase reduce HIF-signaling, which can reduce angiogenesis and thus tumor progression (61). Treatment of cancer is complicated by the complexities and redundancies in molecular signaling of cancer cells. Thus, targeting tumor metabolism through POX-mediated pathways (Figure 2) may be an effective alternative, since cancer cells may be more susceptible to metabolic stress.

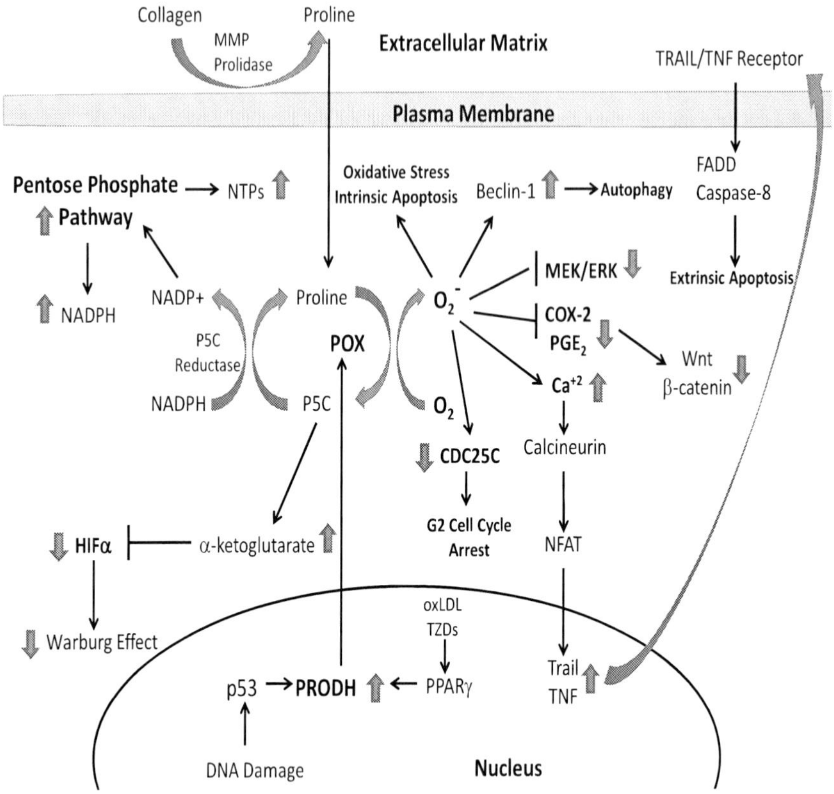

Figure 2. POX-regulated pathways mediating tumor suppression. DNA damage induces p53, which transactivates the PRODH gene to upregulate the POX protein, thus stimulating proline cycling at the mitochondrion. Cycling of proline transfers redox potential to oxygen producing superoxides that can affect numerous pathways involved in survival, death, and cell cycle arrest. Increased proline cycling produces more P5C which produces increased a-ketoglutarate leading to suppression of HIF and the Warburg effect. P5C reductase completes the proline cycle and provides increased NADP+, which stimulates increased production of ribonucleotides such as ATP. Release of proline from collagen in the extracellular environment can provide for a microenvironmental stress sensor.

References

[1] Adams, E. (1970) Metabolism of proline and of hydroxyproline, *Int Rev Connect Tissue Res 5*, 1-91.

[2] Adams, E., and Frank, L. (1980) Metabolism of proline and the hydroxyprolines, *Annu Rev Biochem 49*, 1005-1061.

[3] Dixit, S. N., Seyer, J. M., and Kang, A. H. (1977) Covalent structure of collagen: amino-acid sequence of chymotryptic peptides from the carboxyl-terminal region of alpha2-CB3 of chick-skin collagen, *Eur J Biochem 81*, 599-607.

[4] Hu, C. A., Bart Williams, D., Zhaorigetu, S., Khalil, S., Wan, G., and Valle, D. (2008) Functional genomics and SNP analysis of human genes encoding proline metabolic enzymes, *Amino Acids 35*, 655-664.

[5] Phang, J. M. (1985) The regulatory functions of proline and pyrroline-5-carboxylic acid, *Curr Top Cell Regul 25*, 91-132.

[6] Phang, J. M., Pandhare, J., and Liu, Y. (2008) The metabolism of proline as microenvironmental stress substrate, *J Nutr 138*, 2008S-2015S.

[7] Hu, C. A., Phang, J. M., and Valle, D. (2008) Proline metabolism in health and disease. Preface, *Amino Acids 35*, 651-652.

[8] Phang JM, H. C., Valle D., (Ed.) (2001) *Disorders of proline and hydroxyproline metabolism*, McGraw Hill Press, New York.

[9] Phang, J. M., and Liu, W. (2012) Proline metabolism and cancer, *Front Biosci 17*, 1835-1845.

[10] Phang, J. M., Liu, W., and Zabirnyk, O. (2010) Proline metabolism and microenvironmental stress, *Annu Rev Nutr 30*, 441-463.

[11] Kowaloff, E. M., Phang, J. M., Granger, A. S., and Downing, S. J. (1977) Regulation of proline oxidase activity by lactate, *Proc Natl Acad Sci U S A 74*, 5368-5371.

[12] Liu, Y., Borchert, G. L., Surazynski, A., and Phang, J. M. (2008) Proline oxidase, a p53-induced gene, targets COX-2/PGE2 signaling to induce apoptosis and inhibit tumor growth in colorectal cancers, *Oncogene 27*, 6729-6737.

[13] Liu, Y., Fiskum, G., and Schubert, D. (2002) Generation of reactive oxygen species by the mitochondrial electron transport chain, *J Neurochem 80*, 780-787.

[14] Hagedorn, C. H., and Phang, J. M. (1983) Transfer of reducing equivalents into mitochondria by the interconversions of proline and delta 1-pyrroline-5-carboxylate, *Arch Biochem Biophys 225*, 95-101.

[15] Donald, S. P., Sun, X. Y., Hu, C. A., Yu, J., Mei, J. M., Valle, D., and Phang, J. M. (2001) Proline oxidase, encoded by p53-induced gene-6, catalyzes the generation of proline-dependent reactive oxygen species, *Cancer Res 61*, 1810-1815.

[16] Liu, Y., Borchert, G. L., Donald, S. P., Surazynski, A., Hu, C. A., Weydert, C. J., Oberley, L. W., and Phang, J. M. (2005) MnSOD inhibits proline

oxidase-induced apoptosis in colorectal cancer cells, *Carcinogenesis 26*, 1335-1342.

[17] Pandhare, J., Cooper, S. K., and Phang, J. M. (2006) Proline oxidase, a proapoptotic gene, is induced by troglitazone: evidence for both peroxisome proliferator-activated receptor gamma-dependent and -independent mechanisms, *J Biol Chem 281*, 2044-2052.

[18] Polyak, K., Xia, Y., Zweier, J. L., Kinzler, K. W., and Vogelstein, B. (1997) A model for p53-induced apoptosis, *Nature 389*, 300-305.

[19] Hu, C. A., Donald, S. P., Yu, J., Lin, W. W., Liu, Z., Steel, G., Obie, C., Valle, D., and Phang, J. M. (2007) Overexpression of proline oxidase induces proline-dependent and mitochondria-mediated apoptosis, *Mol Cell Biochem 295*, 85-92.

[20] Liu, Y., Borchert, G. L., Donald, S. P., Diwan, B. A., Anver, M., and Phang, J. M. (2009) Proline oxidase functions as a mitochondrial tumor suppressor in human cancers, *Cancer Res 69*, 6414-6422.

[21] Liu, Y., Borchert, G. L., Surazynski, A., Hu, C. A., and Phang, J. M. (2006) Proline oxidase activates both intrinsic and extrinsic pathways for apoptosis: the role of ROS/superoxides, NFAT and MEK/ERK signaling, *Oncogene 25*, 5640-5647.

[22] Maxwell, S. A., and Davis, G. E. (2000) Differential gene expression in p53-mediated apoptosis-resistant vs. apoptosis-sensitive tumor cell lines, *Proc Natl Acad Sci U S A 97*, 13009-13014.

[23] Maxwell, S. A., and Rivera, A. (2003) Proline oxidase induces apoptosis in tumor cells, and its expression is frequently absent or reduced in renal carcinomas, *J Biol Chem 278*, 9784-9789.

[24] Rivera, A., and Maxwell, S. A. (2005) The p53-induced gene-6 (proline oxidase) mediates apoptosis through a calcineurin-dependent pathway, *J Biol Chem 280*, 29346-29354.

[25] Phang, J. M., Yeh, G. C., and Hagedorn, C. H. (1981) The intercellular proline cycle, *Life Sci 28*, 53-58.

[26] Phang, J. M., Downing, S. J., and Yeh, G. C. (1980) Linkage of the HMP pathway to ATP generation by the proline cycle, *Biochem Biophys Res Commun 93*, 462-470.

[27] Hagedorn, C. H., and Phang, J. M. (1986) Catalytic transfer of hydride ions from NADPH to oxygen by the interconversions of proline and delta 1-pyrroline-5-carboxylate, *Arch Biochem Biophys 248*, 166-174.

[28] Phang, J. M., Donald, S. P., Pandhare, J., and Liu, Y. (2008) The metabolism of proline, a stress substrate, modulates carcinogenic pathways, *Amino Acids 35*, 681-690.

[29] Yeh, G. C., and Phang, J. M. (1988) Stimulation of phosphoribosyl pyrophosphate and purine nucleotide production by pyrroline 5-carboxylate in human erythrocytes, *J Biol Chem 263*, 13083-13089.

[30] Liu, W., Zabirnyk, O., Wang, H., Shiao, Y. H., Nickerson, M. L., Khalil, S., Anderson, L. M., Perantoni, A. O., and Phang, J. M. (2010) miR-23b targets proline oxidase, a novel tumor suppressor protein in renal cancer, *Oncogene 29*, 4914-4924.

[31] Lorans, G., and Phang, J. M. (1981) Proline synthesis and redox regulation: differential functions of pyrroline-5-carboxylate reductase in human lymphoblastoid cell lines, *Biochem Biophys Res Commun 101*, 1018-1025.

[32] Pandhare, J., Donald, S. P., Cooper, S. K., and Phang, J. M. (2009) Regulation and function of proline oxidase under nutrient stress, *J Cell Biochem 107*, 759-768.

[33] Smith, R. J., and Phang, J. M. (1978) Proline metabolism in cartilage: the importance of proline biosynthesis, *Metabolism 27*, 685-694.

[34] Bender, H. U., Almashanu, S., Steel, G., Hu, C. A., Lin, W. W., Willis, A., Pulver, A., and Valle, D. (2005) Functional consequences of PRODH missense mutations, *Am J Hum Genet 76*, 409-420.

[35] Liu H., H. S. C., Sobin C., Roos J. L., Galke B. L., Blundell M. L., Lenane M., Robertson B., Mijsman E. M., Rapoport J. L., Gogos J. A., Karayiorgou M. (2002) Genetic variation at the 22q11 PRODH2/DGCR6 locus presents an unusual pattern and increases susceptibility to schizophrenia., *Proc Natl Acad Sci USA 99*, 3717-3722.

[36] McDermid H. E., M. B. E. (2002) Genomic disorders on 22q11, *Am. J Hum Genet 70*, 1077-1088.

[37] Jacquet, H., Raux, G., Thibaut, F., Hecketsweiler, B., Houy, E., Demilly, C., Haouzir, S., Allio, G., Fouldrin, G., Drouin, V., Bou, J., Petit, M., Campion, D., and Frebourg, T. (2002) PRODH mutations and hyperprolinemia in a subset of schizophrenic patients, *Hum Mol Genet 11*, 2243-2249.

[38] Mitsubuchi, H., Nakamura, K., Matsumoto, S., and Endo, F. (2008) Inborn errors of proline metabolism, *J Nutr 138*, 2016S-2020S.

[39] Jacquet H, R. G., Thibaut F, Hecketsweiler B, Houy E, Demilly C, Haouzir S, Allio G, Fouldrin G, Drouin V, Bou J, Petit M, Campion D, Frebourg T. (2002) PRODH mutations and hyperprolinemia in a subset of schizophrenic patients., *Hum Mol Genet 11*, 2243-2249.

[40] Bender H.-U., S. A., G. Steel, C. A. Hu, W. Lin, A. Willis, A. Pulver, D. Valle. (2005) Functional Consequences of PRODH Missense Mutations., *Am J Hum Genet. 76*, 409-420.

[41] Wu, G. (1997) Synthesis of citrulline and arginine from proline in enterocytes of postnatal pigs, *Am J Physiol 272*, G1382-1390.

[42] Wu, G., Bazer, F. W., Hu, J., Johnson, G. A., and Spencer, T. E. (2005) Polyamine synthesis from proline in the developing porcine placenta, *Biol Reprod 72*, 842-850.

[43] Dillon, E. L., Knabe, D. A., and Wu, G. (1999) Lactate inhibits citrulline and arginine synthesis from proline in pig enterocytes, *Am J Physiol 276*, G1079-1086.

[44] Kawabata, Y., Katunuma, N., and Sanada, Y. (1980) Characteristics of proline oxidase in rat tissues, *J Biochem 88*, 281-283.

[45] Kowaloff, E. M., Granger, A. S., and Phang, J. M. (1976) Alterations in proline metabolic enzymes with mammalian development, *Metabolism 25*, 1087-1094.

[46] Meyer, J. (1977) Proline transport in rat liver mitochondria., *Arch Biochem Biophys. 178*, 387-395.

[47] Vogelstein, B., Lane, D., and Levine, A. J. (2000) Surfing the p53 network, *Nature 408*, 307-310.

[48] Vousden, K. H. (2005) Apoptosis. p53 and PUMA: a deadly duo, *Science 309*, 1685-1686.

[49] Vousden, K. H., and Prives, C. (2005) P53 and prognosis: new insights and further complexity, *Cell 120*, 7-10.

[50] Hu, C. A., Khalil, S., Zhaorigetu, S., Liu, Z., Tyler, M., Wan, G., and Valle, D. (2008) Human Delta1-pyrroline-5-carboxylate synthase: function and regulation, *Amino Acids 35*, 665-672.

[51] Maxwell, S. A., and Kochevar, G. J. (2008) Identification of a p53-response element in the promoter of the proline oxidase gene, *Biochem Biophys Res Commun 369*, 308-313.

[52] Shimizu, M., and Moriwaki, H. (2008) Synergistic Effects of PPARgamma Ligands and Retinoids in Cancer Treatment, *PPAR Res 2008*, 181047.

[53] Zabirnyk, O., Liu, W., Khalil, S., Sharma, A., and Phang, J. M. (2010) Oxidized low-density lipoproteins upregulate proline oxidase to initiate ROS-dependent autophagy, *Carcinogenesis 31*, 446-454.

[54] Dang, C. V., and Semenza, G. L. (1999) Oncogenic alterations of metabolism, *Trends Biochem Sci 24*, 68-72.

[55] Fox, C. J., Hammerman, P. S., and Thompson, C. B. (2005) Fuel feeds function: energy metabolism and the T-cell response, *Nat Rev Immunol 5*, 844-852.

[56] Pan, J. G., and Mak, T. W. (2007) Metabolic targeting as an anticancer strategy: dawn of a new era?, *Sci STKE 2007*, pe14.

[57] Deryugina, E. I., and Quigley, J. P. (2006) Matrix metalloproteinases and tumor metastasis, *Cancer Metastasis Rev 25*, 9-34.
[58] Parks, W. C., Wilson, C. L., and Lopez-Boado, Y. S. (2004) Matrix metalloproteinases as modulators of inflammation and innate immunity, *Nat Rev Immunol 4*, 617-629.
[59] Poulalhon, N., Farge, D., Roos, N., Tacheau, C., Neuzillet, C., Michel, L., Mauviel, A., and Verrecchia, F. (2006) Modulation of collagen and MMP-1 gene expression in fibroblasts by the immunosuppressive drug rapamycin. A direct role as an antifibrotic agent?, *J Biol Chem 281*, 33045-33052.
[60] Sun, Y., Wicha, M., and Leopold, W. R. (1999) Regulation of metastasis-related gene expression by p53: a potential clinical implication, *Mol Carcinog 24*, 25-28.
[61] Surazynski, A., Donald, S. P., Cooper, S. K., Whiteside, M. A., Salnikow, K., Liu, Y., and Phang, J. M. (2008) Extracellular matrix and HIF-1 signaling: the role of prolidase, *Int J Cancer 122*, 1435-1440.
[62] Bogeski, I., Kappl, R., Kummerow, C., Gulaboski, R., Hoth, M., and Niemeyer, B. A. (2011) Redox regulation of calcium ion channels: chemical and physiological aspects, *Cell Calcium 50*, 407-423.
[63] Csordas, G., and Hajnoczky, G. (2009) SR/ER-mitochondrial local communication: calcium and ROS, *Biochim Biophys Acta 1787*, 1352-1362.
[64] Li, H., Rao, A., and Hogan, P. G. (2011) Interaction of calcineurin with substrates and targeting proteins, *Trends Cell Biol 21*, 91-103.
[65] Aramburu, J., Rao, A., and Klee, C. B. (2000) Calcineurin: from structure to function, *Curr Top Cell Regul 36*, 237-295.
[66] Crabtree, G. R. (1999) Generic signals and specific outcomes: signaling through Ca2+, calcineurin, and NF-AT, *Cell 96*, 611-614.
[67] Loh, C., Shaw, K. T., Carew, J., Viola, J. P., Luo, C., Perrino, B. A., and Rao, A. (1996) Calcineurin binds the transcription factor NFAT1 and reversibly regulates its activity, *J Biol Chem 271*, 10884-10891.
[68] Bae, Y. S., Oh, H., Rhee, S. G., and Yoo, Y. D. (2011) Regulation of reactive oxygen species generation in cell signaling, *Mol Cells 32*, 491-509.
[69] Verschoor, M. L., Wilson, L. A., and Singh, G. (2010) Mechanisms associated with mitochondrial-generated reactive oxygen species in cancer, *Can J Physiol Pharmacol 88*, 204-219.
[70] Servet, C., Ghelis, T., Richard, L., Zilberstein, A., and Savoure, A. (2012) Proline dehydrogenase: a key enzyme in controlling cellular homeostasis, *Front Biosci 17*, 607-620.

[71] Zorov, D. B., Juhaszova, M., and Sollott, S. J. (2006) Mitochondrial ROS-induced ROS release: an update and review, *Biochim Biophys Acta 1757*, 509-517.

[72] White, T. A., Krishnan, N., Becker, D. F., and Tanner, J. J. (2007) Structure and kinetics of monofunctional proline dehydrogenase from Thermus thermophilus, *J Biol Chem 282*, 14316-14327.

[73] Sayers, T. J. (2011) Targeting the extrinsic apoptosis signaling pathway for cancer therapy, *Cancer Immunol Immunother 60*, 1173-1180.

[74] Wang, T. T., and Jeng, J. (2000) Coordinated regulation of two TRAIL-R2/KILLER/DR5 mRNA isoforms by DNA damaging agents, serum and 17beta-estradiol in human breast cancer cells, *Breast Cancer Res Treat 61*, 87-96.

[75] Montecucco, A., and Biamonti, G. (2007) Cellular response to etoposide treatment, *Cancer Lett 252*, 9-18.

[76] Beck, W. T., Mo, Y. Y., and Bhat, U. G. (2001) Cytotoxic signalling by inhibitors of DNA topoisomerase II, *Biochem Soc Trans 29*, 702-703.

[77] Lowe, S. W., Ruley, H. E., Jacks, T., and Housman, D. E. (1993) p53-dependent apoptosis modulates the cytotoxicity of anticancer agents, *Cell 74*, 957-967.

[78] Tishler, R. B., Calderwood, S. K., Coleman, C. N., and Price, B. D. (1993) Increases in sequence specific DNA binding by p53 following treatment with chemotherapeutic and DNA damaging agents, *Cancer Res 53*, 2212-2216.

[79] Erin, N., Bronson, S. K., and Billingsley, M. L. (2003) Calcium-dependent interaction of calcineurin with Bcl-2 in neuronal tissue, *Neuroscience 117*, 541-555.

[80] Shibasaki, F., Kondo, E., Akagi, T., and McKeon, F. (1997) Suppression of signalling through transcription factor NF-AT by interactions between calcineurin and Bcl-2, *Nature 386*, 728-731.

[81] Wang, H. G., Pathan, N., Ethell, I. M., Krajewski, S., Yamaguchi, Y., Shibasaki, F., McKeon, F., Bobo, T., Franke, T. F., and Reed, J. C. (1999) Ca2+-induced apoptosis through calcineurin dephosphorylation of BAD, *Science 284*, 339-343.

[82] Srivastava, R. K., Sasaki, C. Y., Hardwick, J. M., and Longo, D. L. (1999) Bcl-2-mediated drug resistance: inhibition of apoptosis by blocking nuclear factor of activated T lymphocytes (NFAT)-induced Fas ligand transcription, *J Exp Med 190*, 253-265.

[83] Gualberto, A., Marquez, G., Carballo, M., Youngblood, G. L., Hunt, S. W., 3rd, Baldwin, A. S., and Sobrino, F. (1998) p53 transactivation of the HIV-1

long terminal repeat is blocked by PD 144795, a calcineurin-inhibitor with anti-HIV properties, *J Biol Chem 273*, 7088-7093.

[84] Ikura, M., Osawa, M., and Ames, J. B. (2002) The role of calcium-binding proteins in the control of transcription: structure to function, *Bioessays 24*, 625-636.

[85] Wada, T., and Penninger, J. M. (2004) Mitogen-activated protein kinases in apoptosis regulation, *Oncogene 23*, 2838-2849.

[86] Holmstrom, T. H., Schmitz, I., Soderstrom, T. S., Poukkula, M., Johnson, V. L., Chow, S. C., Krammer, P. H., and Eriksson, J. E. (2000) MAPK/ERK signaling in activated T cells inhibits CD95/Fas-mediated apoptosis downstream of DISC assembly, *EMBO J 19*, 5418-5428.

[87] Tran, S. E., Holmstrom, T. H., Ahonen, M., Kahari, V. M., and Eriksson, J. E. (2001) MAPK/ERK overrides the apoptotic signaling from Fas, TNF, and TRAIL receptors, *J Biol Chem 276*, 16484-16490.

[88] Wilson, D. J., Alessandrini, A., and Budd, R. C. (1999) MEK1 activation rescues Jurkat T cells from Fas-induced apoptosis, *Cell Immunol 194*, 67-77.

[89] Soderstrom, T. S., Poukkula, M., Holmstrom, T. H., Heiskanen, K. M., and Eriksson, J. E. (2002) Mitogen-activated protein kinase/extracellular signal-regulated kinase signaling in activated T cells abrogates TRAIL-induced apoptosis upstream of the mitochondrial amplification loop and caspase-8, *J Immunol 169*, 2851-2860.

[90] Blanquicett, C., Roman, J., and Hart, C. M. (2008) Thiazolidinediones as anti-cancer agents, *Cancer Ther 6*, 25-34.

[91] McAlpine, C. A., Barak, Y., Matise, I., and Cormier, R. T. (2006) Intestinal-specific PPARgamma deficiency enhances tumorigenesis in ApcMin/+ mice, *Int J Cancer 119*, 2339-2346.

[92] Han, S., and Roman, J. (2007) Peroxisome proliferator-activated receptor gamma: a novel target for cancer therapeutics?, *Anticancer Drugs 18*, 237-244.

[93] Govindarajan, R., Ratnasinghe, L., Simmons, D. L., Siegel, E. R., Midathada, M. V., Kim, L., Kim, P. J., Owens, R. J., and Lang, N. P. (2007) Thiazolidinediones and the risk of lung, prostate, and colon cancer in patients with diabetes, *J Clin Oncol 25*, 1476-1481.

[94] Koppenol, W. H., Bounds, P. L., and Dang, C. V. (2011) Otto Warburg's contributions to current concepts of cancer metabolism, *Nat Rev Cancer 11*, 325-337.

[95] Brahimi-Horn, M. C., Bellot, G., and Pouyssegur, J. (2011) Hypoxia and energetic tumour metabolism, *Curr Opin Genet Dev 21*, 67-72.

[96] Tretter, L., and Adam-Vizi, V. (2005) Alpha-ketoglutarate dehydrogenase: a target and generator of oxidative stress, *Philos Trans R Soc Lond B Biol Sci 360*, 2335-2345.

[97] Wang, D., and Dubois, R. N. (2010) The role of COX-2 in intestinal inflammation and colorectal cancer, *Oncogene 29*, 781-788.

[98] Moreira, L., and Castells, A. (2011) Cyclooxygenase as a target for colorectal cancer chemoprevention, *Curr Drug Targets 12*, 1888-1894.

[99] Dixon, D. A. (2004) Dysregulated post-transcriptional control of COX-2 gene expression in cancer, *Curr Pharm Des 10*, 635-646.

[100] Dixon, D. A., Kaplan, C. D., McIntyre, T. M., Zimmerman, G. A., and Prescott, S. M. (2000) Post-transcriptional control of cyclooxygenase-2 gene expression. The role of the 3'-untranslated region, *J Biol Chem 275*, 11750-11757.

[101] Gupta, R. A., and Dubois, R. N. (2001) Colorectal cancer prevention and treatment by inhibition of cyclooxygenase-2, *Nat Rev Cancer 1*, 11-21.

[102] Castellone, M. D., Teramoto, H., Williams, B. O., Druey, K. M., and Gutkind, J. S. (2005) Prostaglandin E2 promotes colon cancer cell growth through a Gs-axin-beta-catenin signaling axis, *Science 310*, 1504-1510.

[103] Dannenberg, A. J., Lippman, S. M., Mann, J. R., Subbaramaiah, K., and DuBois, R. N. (2005) Cyclooxygenase-2 and epidermal growth factor receptor: pharmacologic targets for chemoprevention, *J Clin Oncol 23*, 254-266.

[104] Liu, X., Lazenby, A. J., and Siegal, G. P. (2006) Signal transduction cross-talk during colorectal tumorigenesis, *Adv Anat Pathol 13*, 270-274.

[105] Phang, J. M., Valle, D., and Kowaloff, E. M. (1975) Proline biosynthesis and degradation in mammalian cells and tissue, *Ann Clin Lab Sci 5*, 298-302.

[106] Eggleston, L. V., and Krebs, H. A. (1974) Regulation of the pentose phosphate cycle, *Biochem J 138*, 425-435.

[107] Krebs, H. A., and Eggleston, L. V. (1974) The regulation of the pentose phosphate cycle in rat liver, *Adv Enzyme Regul 12*, 421-434.

[108] Merrill, M. J., Yeh, G. C., and Phang, J. M. (1989) Purified human erythrocyte pyrroline-5-carboxylate reductase. Preferential oxidation of NADPH, *J Biol Chem 264*, 9352-9358.

[109] Gordon, M. N., Mobbs, C. V., and Finch, C. E. (1985) The antiestrogen LY117018 blocks effects of estradiol on pituitary glucose-6-phosphate dehydrogenase specific activity and on serum LH, *Neuroendocrinology 40*, 381-384.

[110] Stark, G. R., and Taylor, W. R. (2006) Control of the G2/M transition, *Mol Biotechnol 32*, 227-248.

[111] Liebermann, D. A., and Hoffman, B. (2008) Gadd45 in stress signaling, *J Mol Signal 3*, 15.

[112] Girgin, C., Tarhan, H., Hekimgil, M., Sezer, A., and Gurel, G. (2001) P53 mutations and other prognostic factors of renal cell carcinoma, *Urol Int 66*, 78-83.

[113] Suzuki, Y., Tamura, G., Satodate, R., and Fujioka, T. (1992) Infrequent mutation of p53 gene in human renal cell carcinoma detected by polymerase chain reaction single-strand conformation polymorphism analysis, *Jpn J Cancer Res 83*, 233-235.

[114] Albini, A., and Sporn, M. B. (2007) The tumour microenvironment as a target for chemoprevention, *Nat Rev Cancer 7*, 139-147.

Index

A

B

C

D

E

F

G

H

I

K

L

M

N

O

P

Q

R

S

T

U

V

W

Y

Z